CREATIVE STRESS MANAGEMENT

The 1-2-3 COPE System

JONATHAN C. SMITH

Department of Psychology
Roosevelt University

Founder and Director
Roosevelt University Stress Institute

PRENTICE HALL, Englewood Cliffs, New Jersey 07632

Library of Congress Cataloging-in-Publication Data

Smith, Jonathan C.
Creative stress management : the 1-2-3 cope system / Jonathan C. Smith
p. cm.
Includes bibliographical references and index.
ISBN 0-13-155805-6
1. Stress management. I. Title.
RA785.S64 1993
155.9′042—dc20 92-10771
CIP

Acquisitions editor: *Susan Brennan*
Editorial/production supervision: *Helen Brennan and Raeia Maes*
Cover design: *Ray Lundgren Graphics, Ltd.*
Prepress buyer: *Kelly Behr*
Manufacturing buyer: *Mary Ann Gloriande*
Editorial Assistant: *Jennie Katsaros*

Printed in the United States of America

10 9 8 7 6 5 4 3 2 1

ISBN 0-13-155805-6

Prentice-Hall International (UK) Limited, *London*
Prentice-Hall of Australia Pty. Limited, *Sydney*
Prentice-Hall Canada Inc., *Toronto*
Prentice-Hall Hispanoamericana, S.A., *Mexico*
Prentice-Hall of India Private Limited, *New Delhi*
Prentice-Hall of Japan, Inc., *Tokyo*
Prentice-Hall of Southeast Asia Pte Ltd., *Singapore*
Editora Prentice-Hall do Brasil, Ltda., *Rio de Janeiro*

To

Karen Thompson and Sharon Kowalski

CONTENTS

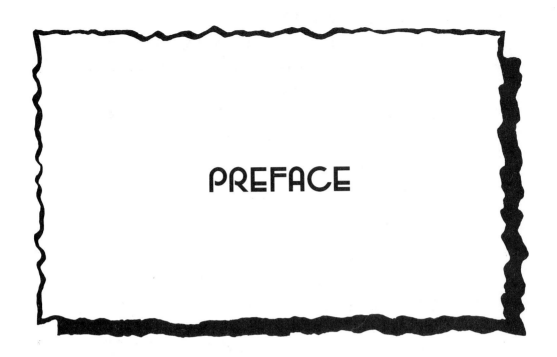

PREFACE

This is a book on stress management. However, it is not a cookbook of answers or techniques. Instead, our goal is to develop *creative resourcefulness*, the general ability to explore a wide variety of coping strategies and effectively apply those that work best. Part I presents a manual of basic problem-solving principles that underlie stress management. Once mastered, this manual can be used as a key to unlock any coping option, whether it be in this book or suggested elsewhere.

Part II offers a comprehensive library of coping strategies, a wealth of ideas for the student and client to explore. Each chapter is self-contained and introduces concrete and practical instructions for a different coping option. Chapters can be covered in any order, combined in a variety of ways, omitted, and supplemented by outside readings. Once again, the goal of this book is to foster a general ability to experiment and explore. In Part III we take a look at general issues related to health, creative coping, and the meaning of it all.

Finally, relaxation is an important component of stress management. Audiocassette instructions for many of the exercises presented in this book are available from Research Press (Smith, 1986).

Jonathan C. Smith

THE FIRST COPING SKILL: THE "PARET" LEARNING AND REMEMBERING SYSTEM

To benefit from any new approach to stress management, you need to learn and remember what you read. Indeed, learning and memory skills are important preliminary coping skills in almost any context.

Many ideas presented in the chapters to come can be applied to enhancing learning and memory. These include time management and procrastination (Chapter 22), managing stressful negative thinking (Chapters 6–9), relaxation (Chapters 10–14), dealing with others who may interrupt your studying (Chapter 16), and even the basic problem-solving perspective central to this book (Chapters 1–5). However, learning and memory are in themselves skills. They are skills that go beyond opening a book, reading, and closing a book.

People often have misperceptions about effective learning and memory. Some think that "effort equals success," that spending a lot of time and energy studying will guarantee that you remember and master material. Unfortunately, much of this effort is wasted. In addition, many students feel it is enough to read and reread a chapter. Here, studying is seen like driving to grandmother's house; if you make the trip frequently enough, you will remember the way. Once again, effective learning and memory are different. Additional myths include:

- You will remember everything you underline in a chapter. I have seen believers in this approach fervently underline *every* word in a chapter. (Underlining by itself does not work, even if you underline a chapter in bright red or day-glow yellow.)
- A relatively recent variation of the above strategy is to *photocopy* every page you want to remember. This is most often used for readings that are in the

library. (Obviously, that which reaches the eyes of a photocopier does not necessarily meet your eyes.)

- If you outline the key points in a chapter, you will remember. (Outlining can be useful, but it is not enough.)
- If you drink enough coffee, you will become so overly alert that you will remember more. (Sorry, this does not work.)
- Study with someone smarter than you. Their success will rub off. (This never worked for me.)

Fortunately, scientists have determined some learning and memory strategies that work (Spache & Berg, 1978; Thomas & Robinson, 1982). And they are so simple that they can be summarized in five letters: PARET (to help you remember, you might think of the "PARET," the misspelled name of a bird known for its ability to learn and remember). It is a system I have found useful in reading any type of material I want to remember, whether it be a college text, a newspaper article, a business report, or contract.

Step P: Preview

The goal of this step is to take a quick glance at a chapter to identify the major topics. This can be done by:

- Reading a beginning summary
- Reading the summary at the end
- Reading headings and subheadings
- Skimming the chapter (reading quickly, focusing on the first sentence of every paragraph).

When you have finished Step P, you should be able to:

Identify in your mind a map or skeleton of the main outline of the chapter.

Steps A → R → E: Ask Questions → Read → Explain

Next, you focus on each major section in the chapter, one at a time. If you cannot identify major sections, repeat Step P. Generally, any section is from one to three pages long. When you have identified the first section, Ask Questions → Read → Explain it.

- **Ask questions.** First, look at the subheadings and key words. Ask questions about them. If you want, write the questions in the margins or on a separate piece of paper. Get involved with your section, almost as if you were talking to a friend. Do not just ask "OK, what does this word mean?" Get creative. Challenge the chapter. Yes, you can even talk back and attack the chapter. If you are having trouble thinking of questions, imagine you are in a class and have been assigned to come up with three questions for every section. Here are some examples of questions applied to this book:

  "1 → 2 → 3 COPE. Is it really only three steps, or is the author trying to fool us into thinking the book is easier than it really is?"

  "OK, just what is 'COPE'? *I* cope by drinking beer. I wonder if the author mentions that."

  "1 → 2 → 3. Does this mean that one has to do three things before beginning to cope?"
- **Read.** This is an obvious stage. Read the section you have identified. Do not read the whole book, just the section you are now considering. Read *actively*, once again, as if you were talking (or even arguing) with a friend. It is OK to underline a few key words or points. However, leave outlining for later.

- **Explain.** You have finished your 1–3 page section. Now stop. See if you can remember the main ideas in the order they were presented. Recite them in your own words, preferably aloud. Better yet, imagine you are explaining this section to a friend who is about to be tested on it (but who has not read it). I have found one of the best ways of remembering material is to explain it to a class. Explaining the material will also reveal what you do not remember. If you have forgotten something, check it and try explaining it again. After you explain a section, you can outline it for future review.

When you have finished A → R → E-ing one section, move on to the next. But remember, don't move on until you can easily explain the section without checking your notes. After all, if you were explaining a section to a friend about to take a test, they would not let you go on to the next section until they are sure they understand what you have said.

Step T: Test You have finished A → R → E-ing every section in the chapter. Now, return and test yourself to see what you remember or have forgotten. You should try to test yourself in several ways:

- Can you outline in your mind the five to nine main points of the chapter?
- Can you look at a list of the terms or concepts introduced and explain it? It is OK at this stage to construct a list of major terms, or to look at terms you have underlined. (Cover up any answers when you are trying to explain.)
- Can you explain how the chapter is organized? What was the logic or theme that guided the author to put the concepts in the order he or she did, rather than some other order?
- Can you read the chapter summary (or introduction) and give a complete explanation of every point?
- Can you explain how different points are connected or interrelated?
- Can you go back to the questions you had earlier and provide answers?
- Can you rank the ideas in the chapter from most important to least? If you were the teacher, which concepts would be most important to test?

Of these steps, reading chapter summaries, reading the chapter itself, and explaining are the most important. In a pinch, you can rely on these.

These steps will increase the likelihood that you will efficiently learn and remember any type of material you read. This is a very useful coping skill that can be applied in many situations in addition to studying at school. Here are some examples:

You are driving through an unfamiliar city. A filling station attendant writes down directions for where you want to go. You want to remember these without having to refer to them in busy traffic.

You have found a very interesting and important article in a magazine. You could copy the magazine, but you want to remember the main points.

Your doctor has given you a pamphlet describing important facts concerning a serious medical condition you have. It is important you remember these facts. You study the brochure in the doctor's office.

You are on your way to an important meeting. Someone hands you a paper and says "read this." Much to your surprise, the paper includes information that will help you very much at the meeting. You decide to memorize it.

Someone is giving a lecture on the radio. You want to remember what they say. You take notes and then apply the PARET method to mastering it.

You are at a business meeting where someone is giving a complicated report. You realize that in about an hour you will have to reply without the benefit of your notes. You take notes and apply the PARET method.

1

WHY LEARN TO COPE?

I have an unusual hobby—collecting stories about stress. These are not tales that appear in novels or soap operas. They are vivid, real-life accounts told by students, friends, and clients. For example, here is a student, Jane:

> I just started college last week. Boy, was I a basket case! I was totally without friends. I wasn't sure what courses to take, and the idea of deciding a major frightened me. To make things worse, I had to start thinking about my future and career. I didn't know what to do!

And here's Rob, a sales representative at a local computer store:

> Work is just too much. People quit without telling me, customers complain, and I take work home because I don't have time to finish things here. I'm so frustrated. Nobody seems to care what I do. And I suffer from headaches and backaches.

And now one more story. Susan has been married for about a year, and is feeling stress:

> I don't know what's going on. My husband doesn't seem to care about things, you know, his responsibilities, my feelings, and so on. Sometimes I feel really ignored and depressed. I don't want to cause trouble by bringing things up. He'll think I don't love him. To make things worse, I am coming down with a cold again.

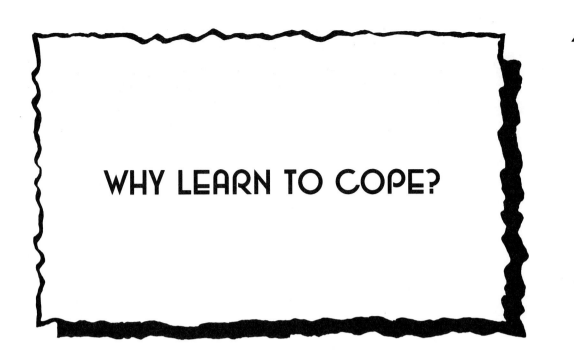

Countless similar stories could be told every day (indeed, I'm sure you could write your own). Such stories illustrate vividly the common sense notion that *stress is wear and tear brought on by demands we can't manage.* This is an important (although incomplete) idea that can motivate us to take the time to learn and try out new ways of solving problems.

Costs of Stress

Most people vaguely understand that stress contributes to wear and tear on our minds and bodies. But the facts make us sit up and take notice. Stress researchers speak of three types of stress-related costs—performance, psychological well-being, and physical health.

Stress, performance, and psychological well-being. Have you ever "gone blank" during an interview or test? Have you ever figured out the most effective coping strategy *after* a stress situation is over? Such problems are common and illustrate that stress can have a costly impact on how well we perform. There are a number of reasons why this is so:

- You have to be awake to do your best. However, too much tension can get in the way. Each type of job you do has an ideal "tension level." It pays to be a little tense when doing hard physical labor. However, some complex tasks, such as writing a term paper or sewing, require a bit more relaxation.
- When you are under too much tension, your attention narrows. You are more likely to get "stuck in a rut," miss complex and subtle details, and think in rigid and oversimplified ways.
- When you are under stress (especially in situations that are unpredictable or uncontrollable), your mind is more likely to become fatigued, interfering with your ability to cope effectively.
- Under stress you may focus less on the task at hand and become preoccupied with distractions, such as body symptoms, catastrophizing thoughts, self-blaming, and thoughts of helplessness.
- Continuous frustrations and coping failures can lead to negative emotions such as feeling sad, irritable, or very angry.
- All of the above factors can also interfere with your ability to work effectively with others. Stress can reduce empathy, helping behavior, and cooperation, while contributing to rigidity, prejudice, and aggression.

Stress and physical health. A great deal of research has focused on the link between stress and loss of physical health. To explore all these links is beyond the scope of this book. However, it is important to note that chronic stress contributes to physical wear and tear and can alter the functioning of the body's disease-fighting immune system. As a result, you become vulnerable to a wide range of threats to health, including:

Allergies
Anxiety
Arthritis
Atherosclerosis
Bruxism
Cancer
Chronic lung disease
Cirrhosis of the liver

Depression
Diabetes
Headaches
Heart palpitations
Hypertension
Influenza
Irritable colon
Kidney impairment

Pneumonia
Skin disorders
Sleep disorders
Strokes
Suicide
Ulcers

Perhaps the most important message underlying the dismal statistics of stress is this: people under stress feel threatened. They feel a gap between what they want and what they can do about it. They feel overwhelmed, confused, and frustrated. They feel, in a word, helpless. However, there is a larger story that has to be told. It is an exciting story filled with hope and promise.

A Revolution of Optimism

At times, pilgrims to religious shrines experience remarkable cures to serious ailments. Why? And why does the placebo, a mere sugar pill with no physically demonstrated benefit, reduce pain as well as aspirin, and even morphine, for 25 percent of the population? Why does a placebo sometimes work for schizophrenia, ulcers, and even an occasional serious case of cancer? There is even a well-known story of a famous writer who was cured of a fatal illness by watching, of all things, episodes of "Candid Camera"? Why? I could add hundreds of apparent miracles that seem to demonstrate some wonderful and mysterious power for managing stress. Science can now tell us something about what this untapped power is.

For the last several years I have been amassing a second collection of stories in addition to those about stress. It is a rather formidable library of hundreds of books and thousands of articles on one topic—coping. One day I stood back and took a thoughtful look at my collection. It became clear that something important is happening in the field of coping today. I like to call it a *revolution of optimism.* As we shall see in a later chapter, the key finding is:

> Successful copers learn to look to the future with optimism (Scheier & Carver, 1987) and hope (Snyder et al. 1991); feel in charge and in control (Bandura, 1982); acquire a sense of "resourcefulness" (Peterson, Seligman, & Vaillant, 1988); and believe in their own capacity to make a difference (Kobasa, Maddi, & Courington, 1981). And these people live longer. They are healthier. They are happier. And they live more productive lives than those mired in helplessness.

Placebos, healing shrines, and yes, even "Candid Camera," may well evoke such healthy "can-do" optimism. It is an optimism that comes from believing that one is not helpless in the face of stress, but that coping options are available.

The harmful effects of stress discussed at the start of this chapter often need not occur. Even when things seem confusing, overwhelming, and frustrating, there is much we can try, much that can work. Indeed, this book might be seen as a manual of optimism. It provides practical instruction for a wealth of coping strategies.

Realistically, no book on coping can claim to be complete. Indeed, to provide some sort of "encyclopedia of stress management" would fundamentally miss the point. However, it is my firm belief that successful coping is the product, not of some special exercise, but of *knowing how to explore and experiment.* This, above all, is the resourceful, optimistic, problem-solving perspective I wish to convey.

How To Use This Book

In this book we will study and practice many approaches to effective coping. Our approach involves the following simple steps:

STEP 1: Get the facts. Many people feel overwhelmed when under stress because they have difficulty trimming a problem down to manageable proportions. We begin by identifying a specific, concrete, and realistic *problem situation*.

STEP 2: Explore and learn a promising coping skill. Our goal, as we have mentioned earlier, is to learn from the revolution of optimism, and to explore the world of coping skills. This book is designed to help you in your explorations. Part I presents a key; Parts II and III, an assortment of many rooms the key can open. These rooms contain a rather unusual library—a large number of the coping skills most frequently talked about by stress experts and clinicians. Each chapter discusses concrete instructions for a different strategy.

STEP 3: Put your coping skills to use—and try again. Once you have mastered a set of coping skills, you are ready to try them out in your problem situation. Don't expect perfection. You may well fail or succeed partially. If so, learn from your mistakes and look for more coping skills to add to your repertoire.

WARNING: ***Stress management can be hazardous to your health.***

What I am about to say made my editor cringe. "Dr. Smith, maybe you shouldn't bring that point up. You do want to sell your book, don't you?" Well, I believe very strongly that it would be irresponsible not to tell you about one important hazard.

There are hundreds of books and thousands of newspaper and magazine articles on stress management. On the positive side, this is perhaps a reflection of the revolution of optimism. There are indeed many approaches for dealing with helplessness, confusion, and frustration. However, what the experts say about such approaches may surprise you. Unfortunately, because of how they are often presented, they most often do not work (Glasgow & Rosen, 1978; Kanfer & Gaelick-Buys, 1991; Lazarus & Folkman, 1984; Roskies, 1983). Worse, they can actually do harm (Rosen, 1982). Specifically, here are the problems:

- Stress management is complex. Different strategies work for different people. Most manuals simply introduce far too few techniques to be genuinely useful.
- Effective stress management must begin with a careful analysis of stress stimulus cues, skill deficiencies, and consequences associated with specific stress situations. Most manuals rely on stress quizzes and tests of questionable value.
- Books often attempt to do too much, and achieve too little. They often try to provide a basic education on stress science and theory while introducing various specific techniques. As a result, neither goal is achieved. If you are interested in stress science and theory, there are some excellent books available (Girdano, Everly, & Dusek, 1990; Lazarus & Folkman, 1984). In your exploration of stress management, it is important to decide if you are looking for knowledge or skills. Do you want to learn about stress or about how to *manage* stress?
- The most serious problem with popular approaches to stress management is that most emphasize the "solo approach." In other words, they describe a

variety of stress management exercises and expect you to try them out by yourself, without the guidance or feedback of others.

One of the basic ideas of this book is that coping skills are best mastered with other people as part of a *coping team*. A coping team can be a university stress management class, a group of clients in counseling, or a self-help group meeting in a local clinic or church. A coping team can consist of two people, for example, you and a friend, spouse, or lover. Even if you choose to explore the world of coping on your own, you can create a coping team whenever you try out your skills on others. The point is to learn and practice stress management skills with others.

Over the years I have become convinced of the value of the coping team approach. When you master coping skills with someone else, a number of very important things happen. You can motivate each other to keep practicing. You can check for mistakes, and reinforce successes. You can challenge each other to stretch and strengthen your coping skills in unexpected ways. You can more easily come up with solutions to tough stress problems (two—or more—heads are better than one). Very often, we are our own worst teachers; it is hard to look at oneself with complete objectivity. As part of a coping team, you can look at stress in a realistic and practical way.

In sum, this is a book on serious stress management. Our goal is to learn coping skills and put them to use. Of course, I cannot guarantee effectiveness; no book can. However, the approaches in this book are based on latest and most powerful scientific principles of stress management (D'Zurilla, 1986; Kanfer & Gaelick-Buys, 1991; Meichenbaum, 1985). We will explore methods that I have used in a wide range of settings, including university classes, clinics, hospitals, and workshops. With this basic map in mind, let us proceed with our adventure into stress and coping.

2

THE FACTS OF STRESS

I like to start coping teams with a puzzle. What do the following stress stories have in common?

- A computer saleswoman has just had an argument with her husband. When driving to work, she is delayed by three traffic jams. At work she makes several simple but serious errors on a report.
- A college student has studied hard for an exam. However, the night before, he learns his mother is sick. While taking the exam, he "blanks out" and simply can't think of the answers to several key questions.
- A college basketball player is preparing for a tournament game. Last month she changed majors, quit her job, left her boyfriend, and moved. Now she is suffering from a sore throat and is worried that she may have the flu.
- A teacher has just had surgery for an ulcer. He worries about catching up with his school work, taking care of his children, and being accused of "goofing around" by taking two weeks off. His recovery from surgery is complicated by unexpected infections.

Each of these stories illustrates the idea of stressful wear and tear we introduced in the previous chapter. However, they also point to another very important idea: there are many causes of stress. Understanding these causes can help make you an informed consumer in the stress management marketplace.

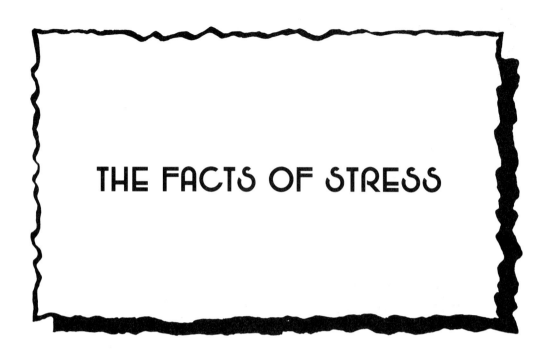

Causes of Stress

The basic facts of stress surround us every day of our lives. Stretching a rope to its limit will cause it to break. A tree blown by the wind will fall. And driving a car without maintenance will send it quickly to the repair shop. It takes little insight to apply such images of wear and tear to human life. Perhaps this is how most people determine if they are under stress. For example, consider the following comments:

"I know I'm under stress—I've got a headache."

"I feel jittery."

"My hands feel cold and sweaty."

"What is stress? It's all the pressures at work."

"These children drive me crazy."

"My school work is just too much."

These common sense notions illustrate the first two causes of stress: the fight or flight arousal response, and stressful life events.

The Fight or Flight Arousal Response

Here are three members of coping teams who have experienced quite different situations. Susan is at the office worrying over a report that was due yesterday. Bill is sitting on the bench getting ready to play football. Chris has just had a flat tire while driving home on a crowded freeway. It may surprise you that each is experiencing the same physical reactions—rapidly beating heart, cold and sweaty palms, increased muscle tension, and a queasy stomach. The reason is the stress arousal response.

Stress arousal is an automatic response developed through years of evolution. It prepares us for vigorous, emergency action through what physiologist Walter Cannon (1929) has called the "fight or flight response." This response is truly automatic. Our ancestors in the wild hardly had time to figure out how to awaken and energize their bodies to fight off an attacking gorilla. However, many of the stress-related problems we experience today can be associated with needless stress arousal.

The number of changes orchestrated in the fight or flight response is truly astounding, as can be seen in Table 2-1. Under stress:

- Fuels, in the form of glucose sugars, fats, and proteins, are released for energy.
- Additional oxygen is breathed in so the fuel can "burn" through metabolism. Breathing rate and volume increases.
- Fuel and oxygen must be efficiently carried to where they are needed—the muscles of the arms and legs that will do the fighting or fleeing. The heart beats more quickly, more blood is pumped with each beat, blood pressure increases, and blood vessels to needed muscles dilate.
- Metabolic rate increases as body fuels are burned. Excess heat is carried away through breathing and perspiration.
- Functions not needed for emergency action are reduced: stomach and intestinal activity are limited, and blood flow to the skin, stomach, and intestines decreases.
- The body prepares itself for possible injury. Surface blood vessels constrict, reducing the possibility of serious blood loss. Clotting substances are dumped

TABLE 2-1 What happens in stress arousal

Organ/Substance	*What Happens*	*Some Resulting Symptoms*
Liver	Releases extra sugar (glucose) to fuel muscles	Increased energy level; eventual fatigue
Hormones	Are released to stimulate conversion of fats and proteins to sugar	Increased energy level; eventual fatigue
Endorphins	Are secreted by brain as natural painkillers	Increased ability to tolerate pain in extreme situations
Fats	Are released and broken down	Increased energy level; eventual fatigue
Glucose	Is released and broken down	Increased energy level; eventual fatigue
Heart	Increases rate and force of each beat; increases blood pressure to hasten flow of sugars and oxygen to needed muscles	Rapid, pounding heartbeat; possible irregular heartbeat
Lungs	Increase breathing rate along with dilation of bronchi, or breathing passages, to bring in increased air	Panting, yawning, sighing, irregular breathing or breathlessness
Skeletal Muscles (Arms, legs, face, etc.)	Grow tense, increase breakdown of food supplies to glucose sugar for immediate action	Muscle tightness, restlessness, feeling jittery, cramps, backache, twitches
Digestive System	Curtails "nonessential" activity	Queasiness, nausea, stomach problems
Salivary Glands	Dry up mucus and saliva (nonessentials)	"Dry mouth," cough, sore throat
Skin	Decreases "nonessential" blood flow	Cold, clammy hands, increased skin problems
Blood	Releases more "clotting substances" to reduce dangerous blood loss from injury and to hasten healing; produces more white blood corpuscles to hasten healing	Easier formation of scar tissue, increased likelihood of allergic response

into the blood stream, easing the formation of protective scar tissue. The immune system increases activity in anticipation of possible infection, or reduces activity to minimize the potentially damaging effects of overinfection and to conserve resources for fighting and fleeing.

- Natural pain killers, *endorphins*, are released by the brain, to help us keep on going in the face of considerable discomfort.
- And finally, the body readies itself for active involvement with the outside world. Muscles tighten, pupils of the eye enlarge to let in more light and enhance vision, palms and feet become moist to increase grip and traction when running, and brain activity increases.

Life Events and Hassles

There is a serious problem in thinking of stress only in terms of the fight or flight response. This is illustrated by one member of a coping team I was leading, a business executive seriously concerned about his health. One evening he went alone to the movies. During the show he noticed his heart beating rapidly. Convinced he was having a heart attack, he rushed out of the theater and ran three blocks to the nearest cab. His heart was beating even more. Then it dawned on him that the movie, one of the gory *Friday the 13th* series, was truly frightening. No wonder his heart was beating quickly! The subsequent panic reaction and cab chase aggravated the situation, but obviously he wasn't having a heart attack—otherwise he couldn't have jogged three blocks at top speed!

The message of this story is simple: you can't always tell from your physical response whether you are under stress, or simply aroused from working hard, laughing, or even making love. A well known stress expert, Hans Selye, hinted at this problem decades ago. He suggested that there are two types of stress arousal: *distress* and *eustress*. Distress is potentially harmful, whereas eustress is challenging, energizing, and contributes to growth. How can you tell if your arousal is destructive or constructive, or if you are experiencing distress or eustress? We need to look at the events that are happening in your life.

One view of stress has become so popular that it has appeared in hundreds of magazines and Sunday newspaper supplements. It has generated more scientific studies (over one thousand) than any other approach to analyze stress. In the 1960s, physicians Thomas Holmes and Richard Rahe developed a simple stress test, the *Life Events Scale*, also known officially as the *Social Readjustment Rating Scale* (See Table 2-2).

The Life Events Scale is an easy test to take. All you do is add up points for all the changes in life you experienced over the last six months (sometimes a year). Thus, if you experienced marriage (50 points), business readjustment (39 points), foreclosure of mortgage (30 points), and vacation (13 points), your score would be 132. This number presumably represents the amount of change or readjustment you experienced.

The Life Events Scale became widely used when researchers found a consistent relationship between the amount of life changes reported and subsequent illness. More than half of those with life change scores from 200 to 300 had health problems the following year, whereas 79 percent of those with scores over 300 became ill. Holmes and Rahe hypothesized that adaptation to change, even positive events, has a cost. Resistance to illness is reduced and the body is subjected to wear and tear.

Life events research gives us some clues as to which situations may be more likely to create stress. Major, undesirable events (loss of job, illness, foreclosure of mortgage) are more likely to create stress. In addition, a cluster of many events can increase stress. And the extent to which you cannot predict the outcome of, or control the course of, an event can enhance its stressfulness (Thoits, 1983). Finally, everyday hassles, although not major life events, can add up and have a damaging impact.

For years, the Life Events Scale dominated the field of stress and the popular press (even to the point where Los Angeles newspapers were advising drivers with life change scores over 300 not to drive the hectic LA freeways to work). However, it does not tell the entire story of stress. Once you compare your stress problems with others, it may become clear that not everyone finds the same life events and hassles equally stressful. Not everyone gets upset over driving a hectic freeway. To understand, we need to look at stress in a different way.

A New Way of Looking at Stress: Thinking and Coping

In spite of the immense popularity of the Life Events Scale, there are problems. It may surprise you that this fact is frequently discovered by coping team participants with whom I have worked. Beginning team members often blame outside situations. They say things like:

"I'm upset with my marriage. My wife is an impossible person."

"School is causing me stress. All these professors are just too severe in their grading."

"Why do I always get into arguments? Why is it people always want to cause trouble for me?"

As stress management progresses, these same people begin to realize that their situations are more complicated than they appeared at first. Events

TABLE 2-2 The Social Readjustment Rating Scale

Life Event	*Mean Value Life Change Unit*
1 Death of spouse	100
2 Divorce	73
3 Marital separation	65
4 Jail term	63
5 Death of close family member	63
6 Personal injury or illness	53
7 Marriage	50
8 Fired at work	47
9 Marital reconciliation	45
10 Retirement	45
11 Change in health of family member	44
12 Pregnancy	40
13 Sex difficulties	39
14 Gain of new family member	39
15 Business readjustment	39
16 Change in financial state	38
17 Death of close friend	37
18 Change to different line of work	36
19 Change in number of arguments with spouse	35
20 Mortgage over $10,000	31
21 Foreclosure of mortgage or loan	30
22 Change in responsibilities at work	29
23 Son or daughter leaving home	29
24 Trouble with in-laws	29
25 Outstanding personal achievement	28
26 Wife begin or stop work	26
27 Begin or end school	26
28 Change in living conditions	25
29 Revision of personal habits	24
30 Trouble with boss	23
31 Change in work hours or conditions	20
32 Change in residence	20
33 Change in schools	20
34 Change in recreation	19
35 Change in church activities	19
36 Change in social activities	18
37 Mortgage or loan less than $10,000	17
38 Change in sleeping habits	16
39 Change in number of family get-togethers	15
40 Change in eating habits	15
41 Vacation	13
42 Christmas	12
43 Minor violations of the law	11

Sources: Adapted by permission from the *Journal of Psychosomatic Research, 11,* Holmes, T. H., & Rahe, R. H. The social readjustment rating scale (1967). Pergamon Press PLC. p. 216.

Now, which events have you experienced over the last six months? Add up their values. If your score is over 300, some research suggests you may have a higher risk for a stress-related illness. However, remember that your attitude towards these life events can also influence the degree of risk you are under.

are not always to blame; thoughts and actions play an important role in creating stress. This very same point is now recognized by stress researchers; not everyone responds to catastrophes, disasters, or daily hassles in the same way. Some seem to be survivors, and others seem to be especially vulnerable.

Let's see what sense we can make out of the following example of stress:

> Tyrone is taking an important exam. As the professor begins to distribute test forms, Tyrone begins to get anxious. He starts thinking, "I know I'm going to fail this exam! This is going to be the end of the world. I'll never get through school." Not surprisingly, his hands start to tremble and perspire. Fortunately, Tyrone quickly comes to his senses, and takes a deep breath to calm himself down. He carefully thinks, "Now wait. Just keep your mind on each question. First, pick out the easy questions. Then go back and answer the hard ones. Don't get caught up on any one question. This isn't the end of the world, just an important challenge." As Tyrone starts answering the questions, he becomes involved in the task. Briefly, he congratulates himself, "Good. That's more like it. Just answer one question at a time."

We can see very clearly that there are two things that increase or decrease stress for Tyrone—his thoughts and actions. When he thinks, "This is going to be the end of the world," stress increases. If he thinks "Now wait, this is just one exam . . . ," and thinks of a sensible strategy for answering questions, stress decreases. The emphasis on the give and take of thoughts and actions is central to current views of stress.

The most widely accepted definition of psychological stress has been offered by Richard Lazarus (Lazarus & Folkman, 1984):

> Psychological stress is a particular relationship between the person and the environment that is appraised by the person as taxing or exceeding his or her resources and endangering his or her well-being.

There are two ideas underlying this definition. First, stress is determined by the extent to which you think a situation is harmful, threatening, or challenging. In addition, stress is determined by whether you think you have the resources to actively change a problem situation or, if a situation can't be changed, whether you can reduce your pain, frustration, and discomfort. Put simply, you experience stress when you decide, "This is bad for me, and I can't do anything about it."

Stress-Prone Personalities

Stress-prone personalities display general patterns of thinking and coping that often contribute to stress and illness. One of the most important of such patterns is the Type A behavior pattern.

Type A behavior. In the 1970s, cardiologists Friedman and Rosenman (1974) noticed something unusual about the chairs their patients sat on—the fronts were well worn. For some reason, heart patients seemed to be sitting on the edges of their seats. Following this lead, the cardiologists started interviewing patients and their wives. A pattern began to emerge. Cardiac patients appeared to be highly competitive and achievement-oriented. In addition, they had a sense of time urgency and found it difficult to relax. Finally, they appeared to be impatient and angry individuals. Friedman and Rosenman labeled this the "Type A" behavior pattern and hypothesized that it contributed to a pattern of arousal conducive to the development of heart disease. Indeed, research supported this notion.

Recent researchers (Lazarus & Folkman, 1984) have emphasized that "Type A thinking" may well be the key to understanding Type A behavior. For example, Type A's are less likely to be aware of early warning signs of stress such as fatigue (Schlegal, Wellwood, Copps, Gruchow, & Sharratt, 1980). As a result, they are less likely to know when they are pushing themselves too hard and need a rest. Furthermore, Type A's appeared to respond to competitive and stressful tasks with unusually high levels of need to control (Glass, 1977; Wright, Contrada, & Glass, 1985). More recent research has suggested that striving for achievement, competitiveness, and a sense of urgency may not be the crucial components of the Type A pattern. Hostile thinking patterns, whether bottled up or expressed towards others, may be a better predictor of heart disease (Dembroski et al. 1985). Whatever pattern of specific thoughts characterize Type A's, it is clear that they are particularly prone, as Lazarus has suggested, to think of their world as potentially threatening, especially fearing not being totally in control.

Positive, Coping Traits

Another set of personality patterns has been associated with reduced stress and illness. It is beyond the scope of this book to explain them in detail, but they include:

Self-efficacy and *hope*, or confidence, that one can do what is required to cope, and that one's efforts will work (Bandura, 1977, 1982; Snyder et al. 1991);

Hardiness, belief in one's ability to *control* events; *Commitment*, or approaching life with curiosity and a sense of meaningfulness; and feelings of *challenge*, or the expectation that change is normal and stimulates development (Kobasa, Maddi, & Courington, 1981);

Optimism, or positive expectations about the future (Carver, Scheier, & Weintraub, 1989); and

Coherence, or a general orientation that sees life as meaningful and manageable (Antonovsky, 1979).

Over the last decade, an enormous and exciting body of research has suggested that people characterized by self-efficacy, hardiness, optimism, and coherence appear to live longer, happier, and less stressful lives (Friedman, 1990). Indeed, hundreds of inspirational self-help books have proclaimed the "power" of such "positive thinking" and coping. It is my belief that such desirable personality traits are not inborn, but develop as we learn and apply effective coping skills. Lacking such skills can indeed be costly, as we shall see in the following section.

Stress and You

We have now completed something of a "crash course" on stress. We have briefly departed from the practical, problem-solving focus of this book to consider some important facts and theories. At the very least it should be clear that stress can be a complex problem. To understand stress and to begin to cope effectively, it is not enough to be aware of stress arousal or to identify what is stressful about a situation. You need to ask yourself these questions:

"Am I experiencing the stress arousal response?"

"Am I experiencing stressful life events or hassles?"

"Are my thoughts and actions contributing to stress?"

Understanding these questions can help you decide how seriously to take the mastery of coping skills. It can provide cues and warning signs of when to start coping, and indications of when your coping efforts have worked. Understanding the basics of stress is part of the first step of effective coping— "fact gathering."

EXERCISE 2.1 *Stress "Costs" Inventory*

The following inventory can be used as both a test of overall stress, and a measure of the costs associated with any particular stress situation. As a general test, simply check those symptoms and behaviors you typically experience. As a situational stress test, check what you experience before or after a stressful situation. Then add up your points.

Physical Stress Symptoms

- ✔ Heart beating fast, hard, or irregularly
- ___ Breathing in hurried, shallow, or uneven manner
- ___ Muscles feeling tight, tense, or clenched up (furrowing brow, making fist, clenching jaws, etc.)
- ___ Feeling restless and fidgety
- ___ Feeling tense or self-conscious when saying or doing something
- +✔ Perspiring or feeling too warm
- ___ Feeling the need to go to the rest room unnecessarily
- ___ Feeling uncoordinated
- ___ Developing dry mouth
- ✗ ✔ Feeling fatigued
- +✔ Experiencing headaches
- ___ Feeling excessively heavy or physically unfit
- ___ Developing backaches
- ___ Tensing up of shoulders, neck, or back
- ___ Worsening of skin condition (blemishes, oiliness)
- ___ Watering or tearing eyes
- ✔ Developing nervous stomach
- ___ Losing appetite
- ___ OTHER: _____

Stressful Thought and Worry

- ✔ Worrying too much about things that do not really matter
- ✗ ✔ Having difficulty keeping troublesome thoughts out of mind
- ___ Thinking unimportant, bothersome thoughts
- ✔ Having difficulty controlling negative thoughts
- ___ OTHER: _____

Negative Emotions

- +✔ Feeling distressed (discouraged, sad)
- ✗ ✔ Becoming irritated or angry
- ___ Feeling contempt
- ___ Sensing distaste or disgust
- ___ Experiencing shyness
- ___ Feeling fearful

- ___ Sensing anxiety
- ✓ Falling into depression
- ___ OTHER: ___

Stress-Related Performance Problems

- ✗ ✓ Thinking in narrow, rigid ways
- ✗ ✓ Becoming confused
- ___ Becoming disorganized
- ✗ ✓ Feeling overworked
- ___ Losing memory
- ___ Making mistakes
- ✗ ✓ Losing concentration
- ✓ Becoming easily distractible
- ___ Losing creativity
- ___ OTHER: ___

Interpersonal Problems

- ___ Becoming cynical or hostile
- ___ Feeling shy or nonassertive
- ___ Becoming less sensitive to others
- ✓ Having difficulty dealing with other's aggression
- ✗ ✓ Feeling less cooperative
- ✗ ✓ Experiencing conflict with others
- ___ OTHER: ___

Stress-Related Risk Behaviors

- ___ Smoking
- ___ Using alcohol
- ___ Using illegal drugs
- ___ Using prescription drugs for stress problems
- ___ Overeating
- ___ Losing sleep
- ___ OTHER: ___

Type A Behavior

- ✓ Pushing deadlines
- ✗ ✓ Feeling rushed, hurried
- ✗ ✓ Being self-driven
- ✓ Needing always to be in control

Hassles (List everyday events that are irritating or frustrating)

TOTAL: ___

EXERCISE 2.2 *Developing Your Own "Stress Costs Inventory"*

No single stress test can claim to ask all the right questions. Each of us has our own special way of responding to stress. In considering your own stress reactions, it can be useful to invent your own stress costs inventory. Think of those stress reactions you are most likely to display. Borrow ideas from the stress test on the preceding page, or from stress tests you have encountered elsewhere.

Then, list your most important stress reactions in the spaces below (you don't have to fill every space, just as many as you want). Then give each a "stress score" to show the extent you experience(d) the reaction. Use the following key. Finally, add up your scores. This is your TOTAL STRESS SCORE.

Here's how much I experience(d) each of the following:

1 = Not at All
2 = Slightly
3 = Moderately
4 = Very much
5 = Extremely

Your Stress Reactions	Your Score
feeling to warm	3
fatigued	2
headaches	5
trouble some thought out of mind	3
distressed	4
irritated or angry	3
narrow rigid thoughts	3
confused	4
overworked	4
losing concentration	5
less cooperative	3
conflict with others	2
rushed hurried	4
being self driven	5
TOTAL STRESS SCORE	50

Once you list your stress costs, you can rate them again and again. Here are a few of the many creative ways you can use your Stress Costs Inventory.

- *Create a "baseline."* For one week fill out your inventory at the end of each day. Rate how stressful your day was as a whole. This will give a "baseline" you can use when trying a coping strategy in the future. After attempting coping strategies described later in this book, do another baseline to see if the strategy made a difference.
- *Measure how well you cope in a specific situation.* Identify a specific problem situation you can encounter at least once a week (studying, taking exams, talking to your boss, dealing with a problem coworker, etc.). Use your stress inventory after each situation to measure your level of stress in the situation. After encountering the situation five or six times, try a coping strategy. Then, take stress measures again to see if the strategy worked.
- *Measure your level of relaxation.* If you choose to learn a relaxation technique from this book, try taking the test before and after each relaxation training session. This should give you some idea of how the technique is working.

3

1→2→3 STRESS

Many people under stress feel helpless, confused, or frustrated. They are not sure what to do or where to go; their problems may seem insolvable. However, it may surprise you to hear that most of these people already possess the first secret of successful coping. This became very clear to me in one very unusual coping team, consisting of a detective, a doctor, and a mechanic. We began by describing our various lines of work. The detective explained how she approached a case:

> Imagine there has been a burglary. The very first thing I do is find out what was stolen, when the burglary took place, who was present, and what they were doing.

A bit later the doctor described how he begins work with a patient:

> I try to obtain a clear description of symptoms. I then ask about what led up to the symptoms, and how the symptoms interfere with work and recreation.

The mechanic proceeded to say how he would begin a car repair:

> Someone brings in a car that isn't working. They usually say it "makes a funny noise" or something vague. What I do is look at the exhaust to see if it is clean, check the engine timing to see if the cylinders are firing, and so on.

These examples have something very simple and very important in common. In just about every aspect of life, the key to understanding and solving a problem involves obtaining *specific*, *concrete*, and *realistic* facts. Exactly the same is true for coping with stress. Our first step is to select a sample problem situation, one that recently illustrates what stress is like for you. Once such a situation has been selected, we can begin collecting facts concerning three "keys" to understanding stress: your coping *problem*, what came *after* the problem, and what came *before* the problem. These comprise the *1-2-3*s of stress.

Selecting a Sample Stress Problem Situation

When people first describe stress problems, they often tell too much. They may seem to be "unloading," "dumping," "getting it off their chests," or complaining about an endless litany of problems. This is understandable. Any stress situation presents a wealth of data. Because such situations are upsetting, it can be useful to begin the process of sorting things out by giving vent to feelings. For example, in one college stress team, George was having problems dealing with people. He really wanted to talk about it, as we can see:

> Everyone seems to want something from me. Why can't people leave me alone? My mother, my professors, my church—they all seem to be saying, "George do this. George do that." Everyone's bugging me!

It looks like George just wanted to complain. It is easy to see why George felt a bit overwhelmed, confused and helpless at first. However, after unloading a problem, it is then time to get down to business. The first step is to identify just one specific, concrete, and realistic situation, a sample of what stress is like for you. Leave other problems for later. Then, imagine you are a lawyer, journalist, or scientist trying to obtain the objective facts about this one situation. Identify:

Who was involved?

What did they say and do?

Where did it happen?

When did it happen?

In sorting out facts, Alec Mackenzie (1972) has suggested the "20–80 rule." That is, 20 percent of the facts concerning a problem account for 80 percent of what is going on. Although this ratio may not fit all situations, it does remind us to look for the specific and concrete facts that matter. To illustrate the first step of describing a stressful situation, let us return to our example of George. After unloading his problem, he was able to focus in on a specific sample situation. His first description of this problem included a number of irrelevant details:

> Yesterday I was studying in my room. My good friend Susan called me up and wanted help on her Spanish paper. Susan means well, but she always seems to be asking me to help her on her homework. Sometimes I just don't want to. And she doesn't return what she borrows. And to make things worse, she doesn't help me on anything. It upsets me that she thinks she can take advantage of me so much. Well, to make a long story short, I agreed to help.

Using the "20–80 rule," George's team noted that a number of facts were not relevant to the specific situation. These include his problem with Susan not returning items and not returning favors. An additional irrelevant detail includes George's opinion that Susan "thinks she can take advantage of me." Trimmed of needless detail, George's specific, concrete, and factual description is much shorter:

> Yesterday I was studying in my room . . . Susan called me up and wanted help on her Spanish paper. I like Susan, but I just didn't want to help. But I went ahead and helped her anyway.

Once you have identified a specific, concrete, and realistic sample stress situation, you can begin examining the three keys of stress.

Three Keys of Stress

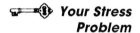

Your Stress Problem

It is the basic philosophy of this book that a stress situation is a problem waiting to be solved (D'Zurilla, 1986). We experience stress when we do not, or cannot, use effective coping strategies to remove a threat or harm, or meet a challenge. Getting the facts about coping with problems involves asking in concrete, specific, and realistic terms: What did I want? and What went wrong? Let's examine these questions in greater detail.

What Did I Want? When thinking about your stress situation, consider your goals. What needs and wants are being frustrated or are in conflict? Most people think of more than one goal. Indeed, it can be useful to *brainstorm* and think of as many possible goals as you can. Your brainstorming rule of thumb is: quantity and variety breed quality (Osborn, 1963). Then after brainstorming, pick the best goal.

People often experience two types of goals in stress problem situations: Sensible or "workable" goals and "unworkable" goals. To return to our ongoing example, George brainstormed a number of goals or "wants" that were not met in his sample stress situation.

"I did not want Susan to call that night."

"I wish I could have politely declined Susan's request without hurting her feelings."

"I would like to find out why Susan wants me to help her so much."

"Boy, I had the urge to tell her to jump in the lake."

"Maybe I shouldn't have answered the phone."

"Why can't Susan be considerate?"

Sensible goals are specific, concrete, factual, and most important, have consequences that, in fact, meet our needs. George decided some of his brainstormed goals were not particularly sensible. "I did not want Susan to call that night" was not realistic. "Why can't Susan be considerate?" was not specific or concrete. "I had the urge to tell her to jump in the lake" was not factual or truthful since George did not really want her to do such a thing. George decided that the sensible goal that was not met, the one that really upset him, was that he did not politely decline Susan's request without hurting her feelings. Since people often have similar trouble identifying goals, here are some more comparisons of goals that do not work and goals that do:

Unworkable Goals *(Vague, Abstract, Unrealistic)*	**Sensible Goals** *(Specific, Concrete, Realistic)*
• I want to be happy.	• I want to ask Joan out tonight.
• I want to be perfect at everything I do.	• I want to do my best on this exam without getting hung up on any question.
• I want to be rich.	• I want to come up with a plan for looking for a job.

What Went Wrong? Once you have identified your goal, look at what you specifically did and thought—at your solutions that did or did not work. Generally, unworkable solutions include *negative behaviors* and *missing behaviors*.

In considering those solutions that didn't work, ask yourself if, realistic, specific and concrete *negative behaviors* interfered with obtaining your goal. Here are some sample negative behaviors:

> Whenever I ask someone out for a date, I put them off by saying, "I suppose you don't want to spend time with a person like me."
>
> Sometimes I need help from my co-worker, but don't ask. I start thinking, "They will think I don't know what I'm doing." These negative thoughts keep me from asking.

In contrast, *missing behaviors* are coping thoughts and actions you could have done but didn't. For example:

> I simply didn't know what to say during my job interview.
>
> I wanted to ask Bill out tonight, but didn't know how to approach him.

We can now return to our stress team example, George. He examined his stress situation specifically, concretely, and realistically. It was clear that both missing and negative behaviors kept him from achieving his goal:

> Obviously, I have trouble saying no. That's my missing behavior.
>
> When someone asks me for help, I start thinking, "Good friends always help. Only selfish people don't help." I guess that's a negative behavior, or thought. It's silly to expect friends to help *all the time*.

What Came After—Costs and Benefits

What are the consequences of negative or missing behaviors that get in the way of sensible goals? It can be useful to look at both *costs* and *benefits*. Costs can include:

- Physical stress symptoms
- Negative emotions
- Worrisome thoughts
- Maladaptive behavior (such as drinking, smoking, taking drugs, or overeating)
- Others' responses to your behavior
- Failure to achieve your goals

Why look for costs? First, if you can see the costs of your negative or missing behaviors, you are more likely to be motivated to change. Second, some costs can serve as cues for future coping problems, as can be seen here:

> After I failed my exam, I started putting myself down for being so lazy. Self put-downs were one of the costs of failing the exam. However, when I started putting myself down, I encountered another problem—I gave up and stopped studying. My self put-downs became a stress cue for my next problem, giving up and not studying.

Negative and missing behaviors can have their payoffs. George, for example, wanted to decline Susan's request for help. But doing so would have been risky and might have made him feel anxious. So he took the easy way out and agreed to help her. This consequence got him off the hook, at least for the time being, and contributed to a pattern of giving in to requests. An unfortunate lesson was reinforced: avoid the discomfort of saying "no" by giving in.

What Came Before—Stress Cues

Most people wait until the last moment before dealing with stress. Then it is often too late to take effective preventive steps. One step in understanding a stress problem is to identify *cues* that indicate that a problem is present. There are two types of cues: *warning signs* and *critical moments.*

A stress warning sign is the earliest indication that there might be a problem, the earliest moment you are aware of potential trouble. It is the weather report warning of a coming storm. George was able to identify his early warning sign:

> I knew I might have a problem when I ran into Susan a week ago. Although she didn't ask for help, just running into her got me worrying. I started thinking, "The semester is just about over. I bet she's going to ask for help soon."

A *critical moment* is that time in a stress situation when the problem has arrived, the time you feel the first raindrop before the thunderstorm. It is the best time to do something. George knew immediately what his critical moment was. He turned to his coping team and explained:

> The moment Susan called, I knew she might ask for help . . . (Then stress began to build).

A critical moment can be indicated by a variety of signals —such as the words and actions of others, your own feelings, your physical symptoms, your own thought, speech and behavior, and your sense of environmental events. Here's a sampling of signals:

When I get a stomachache around my mother, I know things are going badly and we are about to get into an argument.

While talking with my boss, whenever I start thinking, "He must think I'm really helpless," I start forgetting what I want to say.

Whenever my roommate asks me, "Why didn't you go on a date last night?" I start feeling angry and upset.

Whenever the secretary in the next office starts using her noisy typewriter, I can't think and I start making mistakes.

We have now examined all the basic facts of a stress problem situation that need to be gathered. They can be summarized:

CUES → *PROBLEM* → COSTS/BENEFITS

Gathering Facts

Clearly, facts are important for analyzing a situation. Here are five strategies we can consider for fact-gathering:

Microanalysis of a Situation We have performed a *microanalysis* on one stress problem situation. We looked at George's problem in considerable detail, identifying specific, concrete, and factual cues; goals, negative behaviors, and missing behaviors; and costs and benefits. Such a microanalysis can be a useful way of identifying what coping steps need to be taken.

Fantasy A fantasy is similar to microanalysis. Here, you closely go over in your mind every step of a stressful encounter. Identify everything that was done, thought, said, and felt. Imagine you are replaying in slow motion a movie of your situation.

Role-Playing Coping teams can find it particularly useful to act out specific stress situations through role-playing. The simplest strategy is for the person under stress to play him/herself, and for someone else to play other relevant parties. After role-playing, team members can identify cues, goals, missing behaviors, negative behaviors, and costs and benefits.

Diary A diary involves taking notes every day on what stress situations you have encountered. Break your diary down into CUES → *COPING PROBLEM* → COSTS/BENEFITS. Start by outlining a situation. Then, proceed with the details:

Stress Problem Situation Diary for Day: ________________

Situation: (Who was involved? What did they say and do? Where did it happen? When did it happen?)

Warning sign

Critical moment

Coping problem (Goals, missing behaviors, negative behaviors)

Costs/benefits (Negative emotions, physical symptoms, thoughts, behaviors, others' reactions, negative outcome)

Questionnaires Finally, a large number of questionnaires can help you identify cues, problems, costs, and benefits. Some examples are listed below. However, it is beyond the scope of this book to provide instruction in stress assessment, and most of these tools require professional interpretation. If you are working with a teacher or therapist, it is perhaps better to let them decide which tests to use (if any) to supplement the simple exercises presented in this book.

- **Life Events** *The Social Readjustment Rating Scale* (Holmes & Rahe, 1967).
- **Hassles** *The Hassles Scale.* (Kanner et al, 1981).

- **Stressful Thoughts** *Dysfunctional Attitude Scale* (Weissman, 1980); *Irrational Values Scale* (MacDonald & Games, 1972).
- **Stressful Emotions** *Self-Rating Anxiety Scale* (Zung, 1971); *Beck Depression Inventory* (Beck & Beamesderfer, 1974); *State-Trait Anxiety Inventory* (Spielberger, Gorsuch, & Lushene, 1970).
- **Physical Stress Arousal** *The Stress Test* (Smith, 1991).
- **Type A Behavior** *Jenkins Activity Survey* (Jenkins, Rosenman, & Friedman, 1967).
- **Coping Behavior** *The Rathus Assertiveness Schedule* (Rathus, 1973); *Ways of Coping Checklist* (Lazarus & Folkman, 1984).
- **General Stress** *Derogatis Stress Profile.* (Derogatis, 1980).

EXERCISE 3.1 *Describing Situations in Specific, Concrete, and Realistic Terms*

In the space below, describe a stress situation. Remember to include all the details, including:

Who was involved?

What did they say and do?

Where did it happen?

When did it happen?

Now, return to your description. Identify any parts that are not *specific, concrete,* or *realistic.*

If you are in a coping team, have team members discuss which parts are and are not specific, concrete, and realistic.

EXERCISE 3.2 *The Stress Diary*

At the end of each day, describe any stress situations you encountered. First, describe in terms that are concrete, specific, and realistic, the facts of the situation. Then identify **Warning signs**, **Critical moments**, **Coping problems**, **Costs**, and **Benefits**.

Specifics of the situation

Warning signs

Critical moment

Problem

Goal
Missing Behaviors (and thoughts)
Negative Behaviors (and thoughts)

Cost/Benefits

If you are in a coping team, share your stress situations and compare cues, problems, and costs and benefits.

EXERCISE 3.3 *Stress Situations and Your Goals*

Select a stress situation you recently experienced. Identify what goals were not being met. Then describe which goals were sensible, and which did not work.

Situation

Goals

Which goals were sensible? Why?

Which goals did not work? Why?

If you are in a coping team, discuss why certain goals are sensible, and why certain goals do not work.

EXERCISE 3.4 *Role-Playing a Stress Situation*

In this exercise, one team member of a coping team selects a stress situation involving other people. The team member then acts out this situation, he or she playing him/herself, and other team members playing the other people involved. After role-playing, discuss these questions:

1. What were the warning signs for this situation?
2. What were the critical moments for this situation?
3. What were the goals (both those that are sensible and those that did not work?)
4. Were there any missing behaviors?
5. Were there any missing thoughts?
6. Were there any negative behaviors?
7. Were there any negative thoughts?
8. What were the costs and benefits of this stressful situation?

EXERCISE 3.5 *Your Stress Costs Inventory*

Try completing your stress costs inventory (Exercise 2.1 or 2.2) before and after a stress situation you described for this chapter.

What About Hopeless Situations?

Here are some puzzling stress situations that are not that unusual.

Yesterday I broke my arm in an automobile accident. It hurt a great deal and kept me from going to work. There is nothing I could have done about it. Sure, I didn't want a broken arm, but it just happened.

I carefully looked at my finances and have concluded that I am going to have to drop out of school for a year to work. My goal is to stay in school, but there is simply no way of doing that.

My wife and I just decided to get a divorce. Sure, I would like to stay married. But it just wasn't working—for either of us.

Each of these people first described their stress problems as "hopeless." The indicated goals—not having a broken arm, staying in school, remaining married—simply could not be achieved, no matter how sensible the solutions might be. However, a basic premise of this book is that, even though a situation may seem *hopeless*, you are never *helpless*. If you feel helpless, then you have latched onto a goal that is not working. For example, it simply does not make any sense to "wish it weren't so" if you have a broken arm, or have to drop out of school or get a divorce. Through creative brainstorming, you can identify some sensible goals, even for situations that seem hopeless.

This idea can be put a little differently. An overall goal of learning to cope is to replace a *helpless attitude* with a *problem-solving attitude*. Those with a helpless attitude embrace goals and solutions that do not work. The problem-solving attitude is based on the fundamental premise that even the most bleak and desperate stress situations are problems to be solved. The solutions may not be the ones you yearn for in childhood fantasies, but they are solutions just the same.

4

1→2→3 COPE

The most difficult part of coping can be making up your mind. What should you do? When should you do it? How should you do it? Often such difficulties result when we harbor certain attitudes, for example:

"I must choose the perfect solution."

"I don't know when to begin."

"There is only one right answer."

"If I wait, a better solution will come to me."

"It's going to be too painful to take action."

"So what if I try? It won't really change things."

"What if I fail?"

Coping involves taking on a certain *problem-solving attitude* (D'Zurilla, 1986). As we saw in the previous chapter, this can involve taking a hopeless, confusing, and frustrating situation and deciding what coping strategies to employ. Once again, it is useful to examine coping behaviors, as well as what comes before and after.

In this chapter we will look at the *three keys of coping:* (1) What you can do or think in a stressful situation, in other words, your coping alternatives for getting what you want; (2) the costs and benefits of what you might do or think; and (3) the cues indicating when action is called for. In sum, these keys can be put in a simple formula:

WHAT COMES BEFORE → *COPE* → WHAT COMES AFTER

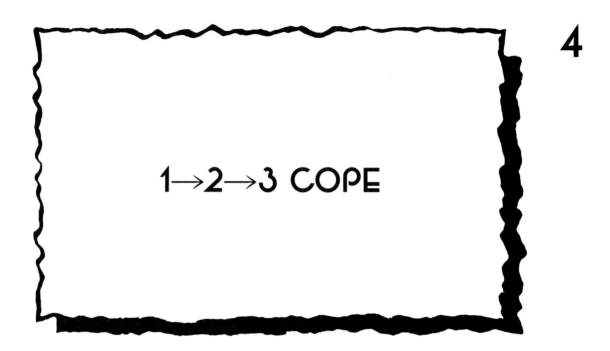

Or, to put it differently:

CUES → *COPE* → COSTS/BENEFITS

Now, let us take a closer look at each of the keys, beginning with coping, and then considering what comes after and before.

Three Keys to Coping

Your Coping Alternatives

Coping includes what you plan to think and do in your stress problem situation. In this chapter we will consider a general way of looking at all coping as problem-solving. Later, in the *Coping library* we will look at some specific techniques and strategies.

As we saw earlier, coping can involve actually trying to change a situation and make things better or attempting to reduce the pain and discomfort of a situation that cannot be changed. In addition, coping can involve avoiding negative thoughts and behaviors that can get in the way, and actually performing missing behaviors that can help you cope.

Goals. Take a second look at your coping goals. What do you want in your stress problem situation? We considered this question earlier when we considered unworkable and sensible goals. However, the goal you first believed caused your stressful problem may not necessarily be the best goal to seek. For example, perhaps seeking a "perfect score" on an exam was a needlessly perfectionistic goal. Maybe, "finding a girlfriend or boyfriend at the dance" was asking too much, or "getting exactly the raise I want" just was not feasible.

One way of making sure your goals are stated in useful terms is to break them into subgoals, and list the steps required for each. For example, instead of saying: "I'm going to work for at least a B on my math exam," you might identify the following subgoals: "How am I going to figure out what is most important to study? How am I going to decide when to study? In each study session, how much should I read, and how much should I review?"

Another problem people often have is conflicting goals. For example, you might think "getting better grades" is a goal and then discover than you have little time to study because you enjoy being with your friends. Here an underlying goal might be "How can I schedule time with my friends and still have time left for study?" Ask yourself why you have selected your goal, and if that is really what you want.

Let's return to George, the example we introduced in the previous chapter. George decided that his stress situation goal, declining Susan's request without hurting her feelings, was not exactly what he wanted. Here is the goal he really wanted to meet:

> I would really like to sit down with Susan and let her know that I like her very much, but that when she asks me for help every week, I feel frustrated.

This goal made sense given his friendship with Susan. In fact, George saw this as an opportunity to work towards a larger goal, getting to know Susan better and deepening his friendships with others.

Coping Thoughts and Behaviors. Earlier we saw that collecting facts about a stress problem situation involves determining negative and missing behaviors. We can now return to your coping problem and think more carefully about the solution. Just as our first goals are at times not the best, our coping ideas are often not the most appropriate. In sorting out your options, it can be helpful to brainstorm alternatives. Remember the object of brainstorming is to put aside your critical thinking cap, and generate as many alternatives as possible. What negative thoughts and behaviors do you want to stop? What missing thoughts and behaviors do you want to employ?

In our example, George brainstormed the following ways of reaching his new goal, sitting down and talking things through with Susan.

> When Susan calls, I could say, "I'm sorry, but I feel uncomfortable helping you today. I would like to get together to talk with you tomorrow."
>
> I could write a detailed letter explaining to Susan what I want to do.
>
> I could catch her in the lunchroom.
>
> I could reply to her request by asking her to do my math assignment for me.
>
> I could quickly change the topic.
>
> I could hang up.
>
> I could promise to help, and not show up.

It might be tempting to consider whatever coping option first seems right. However, you improve your chances of making a good choice if you consider the consequences of your options.

Benefits and Costs

To select your coping option, you need to think about what might happen after you cope. First, anticipate obvious costs that automatically rule out some of your choices either because they pose unacceptable risks or probably would not work. For George, hanging up, changing the topic, promising to help and not showing up seemed obvious poor choices. Next, assess the costs and benefits of the remaining solutions. In weighing these factors, D'Zurilla suggests examining four types of possible consequences: resolution of the problem, generation of good or bad feelings in yourself, costs in term of time and effort, and other costs and benefits. Here is how George evaluated his options.

When Susan calls, I could say, "I'm sorry, but I feel uncomfortable helping you today. I would like to get together to talk with you tomorrow."

Benefits

- I state exactly what I want.
- I get a chance to deal with her feelings in person.

Costs

- It makes me a little anxious being so direct.
- Maybe she'll ask, "Why won't you help me tonight?"

I could write a detailed letter explaining to Susan what I want to do.

Benefits

- Writing a letter would give me time to carefully consider exactly what I want to say.
- It would get her attention, since I never write.

Costs

- Too formal.
- She may not open the letter.

I could catch her in the lunchroom.

Benefits

- Nice and informal.
- We would be in a "neutral place" where both of us feel comfortable.

Costs

- Too public a situation.
- She might be in a hurry to go on to her next class.

I could reply to her request by asking her to do my math assignment for me.

Benefits

- This would let her know what it feels like to be asked for help.
- I wouldn't have to be direct.

Costs

- She might not get the point, and still ask for help.
- She's so smart in math she might make me feel stupid.

After you have considered your possible coping thoughts and behaviors, decide what you would like to do. George decided he would make a date to talk with Susan.

Once you have decided on your coping thoughts and actions, you are not through. A powerful psychological principle is that rewarded behavior is not likely to be forgotten. If you reward your coping successes today, you are more likely to cope successfully in the future. Think of your reward as one final benefit you can select for coping. George decided to take Susan out to a nice dinner after their talk.

Coping Cues

Once you've figured out what to do, you need to decide when to do it. As we saw in the previous chapter, it can be useful to consider two types of cues: *warning signs* and *critical moments.* A warning sign is an early indicator that a problem is brewing. It is also your cue to begin taking preventive steps. In the previous chapter, we saw how George wanted to say no to Susan's request for help on her Spanish paper. Once again, here is his early warning sign:

> I knew I might have a problem when I ran into Susan a week ago. Although she didn't ask for help, just running into her got me worrying.

George decided that this was the time to anticipate a possible request from Susan.

A critical moment can be seen as your key to take immediate action. It is your preselected coping cue as to the best time to do or think of something constructive. We use such thought and action signals every day of our lives. For example, every time you look in a mirror you may automatically adjust your hair or tie; the mirror is an automatic cue. Whenever you eat out, sitting at a table may be a cue for placing a napkin in your lap. And when the server hands you a bill, you begin considering whether to leave a small or large tip.

Critical-moment cues are signals you select beforehand as reminders to put specific coping plans into action. Such cues can be your own negative emotions, thoughts, behaviors, others' actions, or simple environmental events. Here are a few examples of such cues:

> I've been studying for hours and feel *tense and tired*. This is my cue to take a ten-minute break to do breathing relaxation exercises.
>
> My friend has confronted me and asked me to "be a bit more considerate." I'm *feeling confused*. This is my cue to ask for a clarification.
>
> Work is piling up. I've got a jumble of things to do and nothing seems to be getting done. I *feel overwhelmed by my job*. This is my cue to take some time aside for time management.

And George, our continuing example, selected the following critical moment as a coping cue:

"The moment I pick up the phone I realize it is Susan calling."

We can now return to our summary of the steps of coping. As we can see, they are parallel to the steps of stress we considered earlier:

Stress

WHAT COMES BEFORE → *PROBLEM* → WHAT COMES AFTER

⟨or⟩

CUES → *PROBLEM* → COSTS/BENEFITS

Coping

WHAT COMES BEFORE → *COPE* → WHAT COMES AFTER

⟨or⟩

CUES → *COPE* → COSTS/BENEFITS

When to Cope: Variations on a Theme

It is never too early, or too late, to cope. For example, for George an early warning sign was meeting Susan in the street. We can view a warning sign as a stress situation, or coping opportunity, in and of itself. The cue would, of course, be meeting Susan. A coping option might be to put worry aside and talk to Susan. This could be followed by the benefits of George's reduced worrying and the reward of patting himself on the back for facing the situation.

The costs and benefits that come *after* coping can present their own stress situations. For example, after talking to Susan on the phone, George might start ruminating about what he should have said, worrying about Susan's reactions, and so on. He could treat such costs as a stress situation in itself and decide to cope by relaxing and turning attention to his studies. Even the benefits of a stress situation can be cues for future problems. After avoiding talking to Susan (a missing behavior), George may feel relieved of not having to face an unpleasant situation (a BENEFIT). This feeling of relief may prompt him to feel so confident that he may avoid paying his bills (PROBLEM), resulting in fines from creditors (COSTS).

To summarize, there are three variations of our coping formula.

VARIATION 1/*WARNING SIGNS → COPE → COSTS/BENEFITS*

Examples of Useful Warning Sign Cues

The earliest thought "this is a potential problem"

Worry and anticipation about future stress

Negative emotions such as anger, depression, and anxiety

Physical stress symptoms

Problem behaviors, reduced efficiency, rigidity

Increased defensive, aggressive, or nonassertive behavior

The desire to avoid a situation.

Examples of Goals

To anticipate outcomes

To think through what you will have to think, do, and say

To focus on the specific task at hand

To combat self-defeating, irrational thinking

To emphasize planning and preparation

To relax when tension builds

To change that which can be changed, and forget about that which cannot be changed

Examples of Coping Thoughts and Actions

"Specifically, what do I have to do to cope?"

"I can develop a plan."

"I may feel upset, but I can handle it."

"I will just say and do what I have to—there's no need to get too anxious or angry."

"Maybe this anxiety I feel will energize me to do better."

"Let's not take this too seriously."

"Take in a deep breath and relax."

"Easy does it."

"Just stick to the present issues and not get too personally involved."

"Let's not get preoccupied with worry. Worry won't help anything."

"It's OK to feel a little uptight."

"Just keep busy—it's better than getting all upset."

VARIATION 2/*CRITICAL MOMENT → COPE → COSTS/BENEFITS*

Examples of Useful Critical Moment Cues

Recognition that the stress situation is at hand and that now is the best time to do something about it

Worry and anticipation about the situation

Negative emotions such as anger, depression, and anxiety

Physical stress symptoms

Problem behaviors, reduced efficiency, and rigidity

Increased defensive, aggressive, or nonassertive behavior

Examples of Goals

To solve problems and deal with the stress situation

To express what is on your mind

To reassure yourself that you can handle the situation

To reinterpret stress as a constructive challenge, something that could potentially help you grow

To remain focused on the task at hand

Examples of Coping Thoughts and Actions

"I will use this as an opportunity to 'psych myself up' for dealing with stress."

"I will use reason to deal with my fear."

"One step at a time—I can deal with this."

"Let's not get too personally involved."

"Let's take a constructive, problem-solving attitude."

"There are a lot of coping strategies I could use."

"Just 'chunk' this problem into manageable steps."

"Relax and think of alternative courses of action. Then I will make my choice."

"There's no need to make more out of this than is necessary."

"Don't focus on my fear or anxiety, just what I have to do."

"This anxiety (or anger) is normal."

"Let's not exaggerate or catastrophize."

"Take care not to leap to conclusions."

"Try not to blow things out of perspective."

"Look for the positive; don't think negatively."

"Relax. Use my relaxation exercises."

VARIATION 3/*COSTS/BENEFITS → COPE → COSTS/BENEFITS*

Examples of Costs/Benefits Cues

Recognition that the stress situation is essentially over (benefit)

Worry and concern about what has happened (cost)

Negative emotions such as anger, depression, and anxiety (cost)

Physical stress symptoms (cost)

Increased sympathy and attention from others (benefit)

Problem behaviors, reduced efficiency, and increased rigidity (cost)

Increased defensive, aggressive, or nonassertive behavior (cost)

Increased good feeling about yourself (benefit) so that you forget to prepare for the next problem situation

Examples of Goals

To evaluate your problem-solving strategies and identify what worked and what didn't

To find out what you can learn from the experience

To recognize that even small successes are important; to refrain from putting yourself down for gradual progress

To praise yourself for making an attempt to cope

To keep trying; not to expect complete success at once

To avoid putting yourself down for setbacks and failures

To relax

Examples of Coping Thoughts and Actions

"Good. I did OK."

"It wasn't as bad as it could be."

"I made more out of the situation than it was worth."

"I can see some improvement."

"So it didn't work perfectly. I can accept that."

"I can be pleased with my progress."

"Wait till I tell the others how I did."

"Next time I'll do even better."

"No need to exaggerate or take things personally."

"Even if I didn't get what I wanted, I tried."

"I did the right thing."[1]

How to Practice Your Skills

Once you have targeted your desired coping skills, it is time to practice. Two keys to successful practice are:

1. Start small. It is better to begin with easy, nonthreatening behaviors than with complicated problems. If your coping team feels you have taken on an especially difficult task, consider breaking it down into simpler parts.
2. Practice in a safe place. The whole point of practice is to rehearse your coping skills in an environment where it is OK to make and learn from mistakes. A beginning swimmer practices in safe, shallow water; a beginning driver practices out in the country, away from dangerous traffic; beginning boxers practice with safe, soft "dummy" opponents.

Role-Playing One of the most useful ways of trying out a coping skill is with your coping team. In fact, the very role-playing exercises we suggested in the previous chapter for collecting data can be used to try out coping. Several variations of role-playing are possible:

- You play yourself; someone else plays the other party. The rest of your coping team watches and gives feedback.
- You play the other party involved; someone else plays you. By watching someone else "play you," you can acquire additional insight into what you are doing right and wrong.
- You simply watch as other people play you and the other party.

[1]Adapted by permission from: Meichenbaum, D. *Stress inoculation training*, copyright 1985, Elmsford, NY: Pergamon Press PLC, pp. 72–73.

Fantasy You imagine yourself walking through each step of a stress situation, applying your coping skills. After the fantasy, report to others.

Harmless, Real-Life Situations With the help of your coping team, select a harmless version of an actual stress situation to practice your skills. For example, if you have trouble saying no to requests, go to a department store and practice saying no to sales people who try to sell you something. If you have trouble criticizing others, offer a criticism to an anonymous salesperson.

EXERCISE 4.1 *Problem-Solving Test*

Below is a list of some of the behaviors frequently associated with effective problem solving. The more you check, the more you tend to take a productive, problem-solving stance towards stressful situations.

____ I try to see problems as challenges and opportunities for growth.

____ When confronted with a problem, I stop and try to calmly define it in simple, concrete, and realistic terms.

____ In dealing with problems, I try to be open-minded and creatively think of a wide range of ideas before deciding on what to do.

____ When considering several possible answers to problems, I systematically rule out the obvious bad choices, and then weigh the pros and cons of those that remain.

____ After trying to solve a problem, I calmly look back at how my efforts have been successful, and how I might learn from my mistakes.

EXERCISE 4.2 *Thinking About Problem Situations*

Below are a number of definitions of problem situations. See if you can identify what is wrong with the way the problem is defined. For each, provide your own improved definition.

Fault of Definition	Your improved definition	Definition of Problem
		Why does everyone seem not to like me? What am I doing wrong? How can I get people to like me better?
		Whenever I tell my high school students that they should study more, they just don't take me seriously. How can I get them to respect me?
		How can I bribe my daughter to clean her room?
		I have a real problem with my boyfriend. Last night I told him I wanted to be alone and study. He stopped by anyway. We spent the night together and he left the next morning. I wanted to call him up later in the morning to see how he was doing, but he brushed me off, saying, "Don't bother me." I just don't know what to do.
		Not having a job makes me really depressed. I wish I could kick this depression.

EXERCISE 4.3 *A Problem at School*

Think of a problem you have had concerning school. It can be an old problem or one you currently have. Present a definition of this problem using all of the criteria suggested in this chapter. Answer the following questions:

What is the most concrete and specific statement of this problem you can think of?

List all the information relevant to this problem.

Now, return to your list and cross out information that is not particularly helpful.

Define your problem-solving goal concretely, specifically, and realistically.

Define important steps or subgoals needed to achieve what you want.

What are some of the general strategies you might consider?

Brainstorm specific courses of action for each strategy.

Weigh the costs and benefits of each course of action.

EXERCISE 4.4 *A Problem at Work*

Think of a problem you have had concerning work. It can be an old problem or one you currently have. Present a definition of this problem using all of the criteria suggested in this chapter. Answer the following questions:

What is the most concrete and specific statement of this problem you can think of?

List all the information relevant to this problem.

Now, return to your list and cross out information that is not particularly helpful.

Define your problem-solving goal concretely, specifically, and realistically.

Define important steps or subgoals needed to achieve what you want.

What are some of the general strategies you might consider?

Brainstorm specific courses of action for each strategy.

Weigh the costs and benefits of each course of action.

EXERCISE 4.5 *A Problem at Home*

Think of a problem you have had concerning home. It can be an old problem or one you currently have. Present a definition of this problem using all of the criteria suggested in this chapter. Answer the following questions:

What is the most concrete and specific statement of this problem you can think of?

List all the information relevant to this problem.

Now, return to your list and cross out information that is not particularly helpful.

Define your problem-solving goal concretely, specifically, and realistically.

Define important steps or subgoals needed to achieve what you want.

What are some of the general strategies you might consider?

Brainstorm specific courses of action for each strategy.

Weigh the costs and benefits of each course of action.

5

USING YOUR COPING KEYS 1→2→3 REWARD

We have explored the basic keys of understanding stress and coping. It is now time to stand back and consider how to put these keys to use and open, if you will, the "doors" in chapters that follow. The procedure we will suggest may seem a bit unusual. If you are in a stress management class, you may decide to explore this book from cover to cover. Your instructor may choose to skip chapters or introduce supplementary readings.

It is even possible to apply a *browsing strategy*. Indeed, if you think about it, that is how many people explore new coping options in actual life. We can see this in the following stress story:

> Cory has just started college. One week into classes she discovered that she simply did not have enough money to get by that term. She was at an absolute loss as to what to do and was beginning to feel despondent. Cory decided to ask around. Her roommate suggested a part-time job as a clerk in the local department store. Another classmate noted that he saved money one semester by living with his parents. A school counselor described how students could take out a special student loan to get by. Considering all her options, Cory decided she would work as a clerk. This would involve learning the skills of doing store work, and then applying them on the job.

Notice that Cory browsed through a number of options before deciding what to do. You can use a similar strategy with this book:

1. Select your target coping skills.
2. Find the appropriate skill chapter or chapters in this book. At the end of most chapters are exercises you can use to practice your targeted coping skill.
3. Come back to this chapter. Contract to apply the skill learned in a stress situation.

This is actually how we master most new skills in life. If you wanted to learn to dance, you would first target the skill you wanted to master, say modern dancing. You would then find an appropriate teacher or class and learn the basic steps. When you have mastered your dance skills, you can then try them out on a date. Here are the steps described in detail:

Select Your Target Coping Skills

If you have come this far, you have already picked a sample stress situation and identified goals that are not being met. Most important, you have done some thinking about missing and negative thoughts and behaviors. Now is the time to review what you have identified. Think about it. Is your problem behavior a specific instance of a more general type of behavior that is a problem for you? Is it one example of a problem pattern? In our ongoing stress team example, George decided that his difficulty in declining Susan's request for help was a sign of a more general problem of declining requests from nearly anyone. He also wanted to learn how to relax.

Find and Learn the Appropriate Skill Chapter

The second portion of this book consists of a Coping Skills Library. These are summarized in the Coping Catalog printed on tinted pages. At the beginning of each chapter, a target coping skill is identified. This is followed by a brief list of some of the problems for which this skill can be used. Finally, the skill is illustrated in a brief example. It is important to recognize the impossibility of listing all combinations of various coping skills. One of the most useful coping skills you can develop is a sense of flexible resourcefulness, an ability to see how a strategy that worked in one situation may well work in others. That is, even though a coping technique is not applied in an example relevant to you, think creatively and try to imagine how it might be applied. George found two chapters that interested him. Here they are:

CHAPTER 11
PHYSICAL RELAXATION TECHNIQUES

Target Coping Skills

- Three physical relaxation techniques—tensing up and letting go, stretching, and breathing.

Good For

- General relaxation
- Particularly useful for beginners
- Reducing physical arousal symptoms
- Stress preparation (after stress warning sign)
- Stress recovery (at consequence stage)
- Increasing general energy and alertness
- Preparing for sleep
- As "warm-up" preparation for mental relaxation exercise

Example

Jose is a basketball player. Before a game he experiences so much tension that it interferes with his game. He is particularly tense in the shoulders. In addition his breathing is short and forced. He has found several pre-game relaxation exercises to be particularly valuable for reducing excess tension. He tightens up and shrugs his shoulders, and then lets go. Then he stretches his arms and legs out. He completes his relaxation by taking a few deep breaths. At the end, he rewards himself with a good glass of water, and begins the game.

CHAPTER 16
MAKING REQUESTS, SAYING NO, AND DEALING WITH CONFLICT

Target Coping Skills

Effectively stating a request, including the facts and your feelings that make your request one that should be taken seriously; outlining the benefits if your request is met, and the costs if it is not.

Good For

- Asking for raises.
- Saying no to reasonable sounding requests you just don't want to honor (helping friends or relatives, volunteering for community organizations, etc.).
- Asking for someone else to change his or her behavior if it is hurting or offending you.
- Making a request in any difficult interpersonal situation.

Example

Patricia wants to ask her boss for a raise. She has worked well for over three years without a single raise, and feels her contributions to the company are being slighted. The moment she sees her boss, she approaches him and offers a reasonable, adult proposal: "I have worked for this company for over three years and have not received a single raise. This frustrates me since I see others getting raises. I guess my sense of fairness tells me that good performance should be rewarded, and I feel I am performing well. I would like to put in a request for a raise this year. Frankly, getting a raise will make me feel much better about working here and 'going the extra mile' to do a good job." After making the proposal, she praises herself for making such a good presentation.

When reading Chapter 16 on requests, George discovered that negative thinking and worry can often prevent people from being assertive. He then added Chapters 6 and 7, Catching Stressful Thoughts and Changing Stressful Assumptions and Beliefs, to his assignment.

At the end of each chapter, George found a variety of exercises that helped him learn these skills. With his coping team, he practiced. He role-played declining requests from friends, family members, professors, and church members. He practiced this skill in various mental imagery exercises. When he felt he knew his target skills, he returned to this chapter to apply them.

Apply Your skills

Your last task is to return to this chapter. You will write a CUE → COPE → REWARD contract involving your new coping skills. Basically, you contract to apply your COPING SKILL at a predetermined CUE time and REWARD yourself when doing so. Your contract will follow the general formula:

CUE → COPING STRATEGY FROM CHAPTER ______→ REWARD

Your CUE → COPE → REWARD Contract

All too often the road toward successful coping is paved with good intentions but pitted with failures along the way. It is often easy to promise yourself to make a change, but difficult to carry out. A CUE→COPE→REWARD contract is a way of systematically enhancing your chances of success. Here are its basic principles (adapted from Kanfer and Galeick-Buys, 1991):

1. *When will you apply your coping skills*? Decide whether you want to target coping after a warning sign, critical moment, or consequence. Specify target dates for when you will begin and complete your task.
2. *What will you do*? Spell out in specific, concrete, and behavioral terms the exercise or exercises you plan to do. Make your goals limited, simple, and realistic. It is better to attempt one small change rather than a big change.
3. *How and when will you reward yourself*? A crucial part of a contract is a reward you promise yourself upon completion. Pick a reward that fits the task, one that is not too generous or stingy.

Be sure to give yourself a reward immediately after you achieve your goal. State the timing of it in your contract. Write in your immediate and long-term rewards. For example, during the week, you might decide to give yourself a verbal pat on the back every time you do your homework. At the end of the week, if you've completed four evenings of homework, give yourself a bigger, long-term reward.

All rewards are not equal. In your selection, use the following principles (adapted from Nemeroff and Karoly, 1991):

- Pick an appropriate reward. Make sure it is not too big or too small, given your coping goal.
- Pick a reward you can give yourself right after you implement your coping solution. Delayed rewards are less effective.
- Select as your reward something new. (If you have ice cream every evening, do not use ice cream as your reward.)
- When practicing a coping solution, vary your rewards. It is possible to wear a reward out through overuse.
- When practicing a coping solution, first reward yourself after every success. Then be a bit more sparing in your rewards, rewarding every other or every third success.
- Involve other people in your reward plans. Better yet, make other people part of your reward. Tell your coping team what you plan to do. Share your reward (for example, eat dinner with a friend).
- If you cannot think of a reward, you might use the *Premack principle* (Premack, 1959). Put simply, you can use a high-probability behavior (e.g., an activity you already like and do) to reward a lower-probability behavior (your coping solution). For example, if you frequently spend a half hour each evening at your favorite video game, use this high-probability behavior as your reward for successful coping.
- Use simple kindness as a reward, supplemented occasionally with a tangible reinforcement. That is, during the week, reward each coping success with a verbal pat on the back by thinking, "There, I did a good job." Then, at the end of the week, give yourself something, like a dinner or movie.

In addition to the three basic principles just described, you may want to consider the remaining three questions in your contract:

4. *How and when will you penalize yourself for not completing your task? (optional)* Select an appropriate and specific penalty for not completing your specific goal.
5. *What bonuses might you award yourself? (optional)* It is a good idea to include a bonus clause in your contract. Bonuses are special rewards for when you achieve more than you contracted for (or complete your goal before the time stated in your contract).
6. *How will you keep a record?* Most of the exercises in this book involve completing some sort of written assignment. Completion of this task represents a written record (or proof) that you have met your goal. In all contracts, try to set up some type of record-keeping system before you start working toward your goal. Write down the CUES → PROBLEMS → COSTS/BENEFITS for each day. This record will serve as a baseline so you can see exactly the costs of your problem. (See Exercises 2.1 and 2.2 for scales for recording the COSTS of your coping problems.) Your baseline can also enable you to see what changes occur when you implement your CUE → COPE → REWARD plans. You can see how you are succeeding, and how you might do better.

   For example, if your goal is to practice a relaxation exercise twice a day, begin by recording what happens on days you do not practice (using Exercise 2.1 or 2.2). Then, begin and record your practice sessions. When you reach your target of twice a day, give yourself your reward. Whatever system you select, your contract should state explicitly how you will keep records.

Here is how George chose to contract for applying his new coping skills:

When will you apply your coping skills? I've identified a critical moment, when Susan calls, as well as a warning sign, when I run into Susan on the street. I will plan coping strategies for each. I plan to put my coping skills to use sometime in the next three weeks.

What will you do? When Susan calls, I will first take a deep breath and relax. Then I will tell myself, "It is OK to say no to requests from friends. This is not the end of the world." If she asks for help on an assignment, I will answer, "Susan, I feel uncomfortable helping tonight. I would like to get together with you tomorrow for a talk." If I run into Susan on the street (my warning sign), I will also take a deep breath and relax. I won't start worrying. Instead, I'll think, "Susan's my friend. If she calls and asks for help, I know what to do. I can relax."

How and when will you reward yourself? If I actually do this in the next three weeks, I will treat myself and Susan to a good meal out. I will tell my roommate, also a good friend, of my plans beforehand so he can give me moral support.

How and when will you penalize yourself for not completing your task? If I don't complete this plan, I will stay home Thursday night and study, rather than play pool with the guys.

What bonuses might you award yourself? If I have my talk with Susan before she asks for help, I will give myself the bonus of going out to a movie the same night.

How will you keep a record? Well, I've checked off October 3–October 7 in red on my calendar and have left a place to indicate if I talk with Susan. The day I do this, I will put a big red X on my calendar.

What If It Doesn't Work?

Hopefully your contract will enable you to transform a problem situation into a coping success. However, your initial coping attempts may not succeed, leaving you with a problem situation. At this time I recommend that you and your coping team need to take a careful look at what happened. Consider your failed coping attempt as part of a problem. Look at the costs and benefits. Was your attempt a partial success? Were your goals sensible? Should you try a completely different coping strategy, or perhaps combine strategies? You might want to consider relapse prevention (Chapter 25), interfering negative behaviors (Chapter 24), desensitization, or stress inoculation training (Chapter 26). In more general terms, consider a coping failure as a CUE to reconsider your stress situation in terms of Chapters 3, 4, and 5:

COPING FAILURE

↓

WHAT WENT WRONG? (Chapter 3)

↓

WHAT MIGHT YOU TRY NEXT? (Chapter 4)

↓

OK. LET'S TRY ANOTHER COPING STRATEGY (Chapter 5)

Each application of a coping strategy is something of an experiment, not a final test or guaranteed solution. Part of the process of learning to cope is learning the skill of trying out a strategy and, if it doesn't work, trying another. The first strategy you pick may not be the best. You and your coping team may choose to try a variety of solutions, or combine solutions.

Conclusion to Part I

One member of a coping team had a problem after trying to use the 1→2→3 COPE system:

> There are so many steps! I get so bogged down in trying to figure out what I should do that I get lost.

In applying the 1→2→3 COPE system, it is important to keep a sense of perspective. My goal in writing this book is not to create an army of 1→2→3 COPE robots who mechanically apply each step of the system. The first few times you use this system, it may well seem a bit studied and calculated. This is normal, and is what we usually experience when mastering any new skill. Your first steps at dancing, playing tennis, singing, and even learning to walk as a child were deliberate efforts. However, after some practice, 1→2→3 COPE can be as automatic and natural as dancing, playing tennis, singing, and walking.

Perhaps the best sign that you have acquired the skills in this book is how you feel about stress. As we mentioned earlier, the overall goal of this book is to encourage a sense of *creative resourcefulness*, an optimistic, problem-solving attitude. Once you have this sense, the one or two components of the 1→2→3 COPE system you most need will come to mind more or less automatically. In a resourceful frame of mind, you may think:

"Now is the time to break my problem down into manageable proportions."

"Let's see, what do I really want?"

"Let's brainstorm about my specific options."

"I know what to do. Let's see when I should really get to work," and, most important,

"When I get through with this, I really deserve a big reward."

Learning to cope is learning to experiment and try things out. It is even treating a setback in coping as another problem situation, one that calls for its own solutions. With this challenge in mind, let us now consider the many worlds of coping.

EXERCISE 5.1 *Writing a Contract*

In the spaces below, write a COPING contract. Have your coping team (or another person) review what you have written.

1. *When will you apply your coping skills?*

Describe warning sign, if any:

Describe critical moment, if any:

Describe consequence cue, if any:

Target Date:

2. *What will you do?*

Specific goal:

Thoughts and actions:

3. *How and when will you reward yourself?*

4. *How and when will you penalize yourself for not completing your task? (optional)*

5. *What bonuses might you award yourself? (optional)*

6. *How will you keep a record?*

EXERCISE 5.2 *Your Coping Record*

This chart will enable you to keep an ongoing record of your coping experiments. You can record what you did, what happened, what worked, what didn't work, how you might improve your coping strategies in the future, and how you might combine exercises.

Date	*Cue*	*Coping Strategy*	*Reward*	*What Happened*	*What Worked*	*What Didn't Work*	*Improvements Combinations*

A COPING CATALOG

The remainder of this book contains instructions for a wide variety of coping strategies. These are summarized in the following Coping Catalog. Browse through this catalog, just as you might browse through a library or bookstore. When you find a summary of a coping strategy that seems interesting, you can turn to the chapter that presents complete instructions.

Stressful Thinking and Worry

Is stress all in the mind? Although this idea is oversimplified, much stress is created by stressful thinking and worry. In Chapters 6–9 we will learn how to identify such thoughts, change them, stop them, and how to explore hidden thoughts and feelings that may be contributing to stress.

Chapter 6 Catching Stressful Thoughts

Target Coping Skills

- Identifying maladaptive, irrational thinking that contributes to needless stress

Purpose

- Stressful worry
- Most stress situations

Example

Bruce tends to make bad situations worse, but he isn't quite sure how this happens. Others have told him that thoughts can contribute to stress, but he is not aware of how his thoughts may be doing this. For a week he completes a special "thought catching" exercise that involves taking notes of what is going through his mind right after he notices he has encountered a stressful situation. When he remembers to do this, he says "good" to himself. Bruce soon discovers he creates needless stress by catastrophizing, that is, making mountains out of molehills. CUE → COPE → REWARD summary: STRESSFUL SITUATION → THOUGHT CATCHING → SAYING "GOOD" TO SELF

Chapter 7 Changing Stressful Assumptions and Beliefs

Target Coping Skills

- Replacing irrational and useless thoughts with rational and productive thoughts

Purpose

- Reduction of worry
- Coping with most stressful situations

Example

Ann shares a desk with another worker, Sally. Unfortunately, Sally does not put her things away and leaves a mess for Ann to tidy up. This upsets Ann considerably, but she is having a hard time confronting Sally. A number of negative thoughts get in the way, including: "I can't criticize Sally, she might think I'm too picky." In exploring this thought, Ann discovered it was part of a more general belief: "If you want people to like you, don't criticize." In her coping team, Ann carefully analyzed this belief and decided it was not rational or useful. She decided it would be much better to think,"Good friends can be frank with each other." This change of thinking was praised by her coping team. CUE → COPE → REWARD summary: NEGATIVE IRRATIONAL BELIEF → ANALYSIS OF BELIEF / REPLACEMENT WITH MORE RATIONAL AND USEFUL BELIEF → TEAM PRAISE

Chapter 8 Reducing Worry

Target Coping Skills

- Temporarily stopping needless worry

Purpose

- Supplementing techniques for reducing stressful thinking

Example

John has been trying to change his stressful thinking patterns. He is fairly good at identifying when his thoughts are needlessly stressful, and he can even think of alternatives for his stressful thoughts that are more reasonable. However, he needs a little "booster," something to help him break the pattern of obsessive negative rumination. He tries a simple exercise that involves thinking the word "STOP!" with considerable emotional intensity whenever he starts ruminating. He then does a pleasurable relaxation exercise and goes on working. CUE → COPE → REWARD summary: OBSESSIVE THINKING → THINKING "STOP!" → PLEASURABLE RELAXATION

Chapter 9 Getting in Touch with Yourself

Target Coping Skills

- Uncovering hidden thoughts and feelings; exploring why you are really upset, depressed, confused or anxious

Purpose

- Clarification of reasons for wanting to attempt a coping skill
- Identification of goals
- Preparation for brainstorming coping options
- Release of pent-up emotions

Example

Cynthia is starting college. Although she had planned to live on campus, financial problems are forcing her to live at home. She is alone in her room and feeling confused and "down in the dumps." Cynthia has spent hours trying to figure out why she feels so bad, but with no success. She decides to try a focusing exercise that has helped her in the past. First she sits down and makes herself comfortable. Then she lets her mind become quiet, and puts aside attempts to think about or figure out her problem. She quietly attends to her feeling of being "down in the dumps," and asks, "What is the main thing about this feeling?" Without trying to figure things out, she waits. A variety of thoughts come and go that do nothing to clarify the causes. Suddenly she has a thought that fits perfectly what she is feeling: "I don't want to live with my parents! I feel trapped! I want to live on my own!" After finishing the exercise, she treats herself with a good taco. CUE → COPE → REWARD summary: FEELING "DOWN IN THE DUMPS" → FOCUSING EXERCISE → TACO TREAT

Relaxation

Relaxation can be a powerful way of reducing potentially dangerous stress arousal, as well as preparing for and recoving from stress. Different techniques work for different people. We will consider the most widely used forms of passive relaxation: isometric squeeze relaxation, yoga stretching, breathing, thematic imagery, and meditation. In addition, we will look at some specialized techniques and how to make your own relaxation program. If you are seriously interested in learning relaxation, it would be a good idea to try all of the techniques mentioned in Chapters 10–14.

Chapter 10 Taking Time Off as a Relaxation Exercise

Target Coping Skills

- Learning to set time aside every day for a relaxing activity

Purpose

- General relaxation
- Preparation for physical or mental relaxation training

Example

Rosemary lives a hectic life. Not only is she an administrative assistant in a major university, but she volunteers for several charitable organizations and works for her local hospital. She wanted to do something simple to reduce tension at the end of the day. Using the ideas in this chapter, she scheduled a 30-minute period after work to read for pleasure. Rosemary was surprised how effective this simple exercise was, and congratulated herself for sticking with the schedule. Perhaps it worked because her time-off period became a "healthy habit," a sacred time that could not be touched. Perhaps it provided a useful period for self-nurturing and taking care of her own needs, rather than worrying about others. CUE → COPE → REWARD summary: END OF WORK → PLEASURE READING → CONGRATULATIONS

Chapter 11 Practicing Physical Relaxation Techniques

Target Coping Skills

- Three physical relaxation techniques—tensing up and letting go, stretching, and breathing

Purpose

- General relaxation
- Particular usefulness for beginners
- Reduction of physical arousal symptoms
- Stress preparation (after stress warning sign)
- Stress recovery (at consequence stage)
- Increase in general energy and alertness
- Preparation for sleep
- "Warm-up" preparation for mental relaxation exercise

Example

Jose is a basketball player. Before a game he experiences so much tension that it interferes with his game. He is particularly tense in the shoulders. In addition, his breathing is short and forced. He has found several pre-game relaxation exercises to be particularly valuable for reducing excess tension. He tightens up and shrugs his shoulders, and then lets go. Then he stretches his arms and legs out. He completes his relaxation by taking a few deep breaths. At the end, he rewards himself with a good glass of water, and begins the game. CUE → COPE → REWARD summary: PRE-GAME TENSION → RELAXATION EXERCISES → GLASS OF WATER

Chapter 12 Practicing Mental Relaxation

Target Coping Skills

- Thematic imagery, fantasizing, visualizing
- Meditating

Purpose

- General relaxation
- Alleviation of worry
- Self-exploration
- Reduction of physical arousal symptoms
- Stress preparation (after stress warning sign)
- Stress recovery (at consequence stage)
- Increased general energy and alertness
- Preparation for sleep

Example

Beth has tried physical relaxation techniques without success. She finds them frustrating and a bit boring. She does like to relax by engaging in a pleasant fantasy, or going off by herself to a quiet place. Recently she learned imagery and meditation in a stress management class, and seems to like what these techniques offer. Before breakfast, she takes a 20-minute fantasy/relaxation break. Breakfast becomes a pleasant reward. CUE → COPE → REWARD summary: WAKING UP → FANTASY/RELAXATION → BREAKFAST

Chapter 13 Using Specialized Relaxation Strategies

Target Coping Skills

- Practicing self-suggestion to relax
- Shortening relaxation

Purpose

- Development of brief relaxation strategies for special situations
- Detection of relaxing activities in everyday life
- Overcoming difficulties in learning to relax

Example

Bill is having some trouble learning relaxation. When he tries a technique, he gets distracted and finds it hard to continue, yet he wants very much to enhance his ability to relax. In this lesson he learned three useful tools. First, he identified everyday activities he already does that are forms of relaxation. He discovered that he can become deeply relaxed after 30 minutes of jogging, so he carefully schedules a jogging session at 5:00 P.M. every other day. After jogging, he indulges in a good shower. In addition, he sought the assistance of a health professional to learn the use of special biofeedback equipment to help him determine when he is most tense and most relaxed. Finally, he learned some very brief relaxation exercises that can be practiced on the bus or at work. CUE → COPE → REWARD summary: 5:00 P.M. → JOGGING → A GOOD SHOWER

Chapter 14 Making a Relaxation Script or Tape

Target Coping Skills

- Combining favorite relaxation exercises for a specific relaxation goal
- Making a relaxation tape

Purpose

- Advanced relaxation for those who have already mastered more than one relaxation technique
- Any relaxation goal, including managing stress, combating insomnia, waking up refreshed in the morning, enhancing creativity and productivity, enhancing personal growth and exploration

Example

Sheila has spent many years exploring the relaxation marketplace. She has tried yoga, self-hypnosis, meditation, and a variety of relaxation tapes. However, none seems just right for her relaxation goals. She wants a brief exercise to use whenever her shoulders begin to feel tense—an early-warning stress cue. Using the exercises in this chapter, she made her own relaxation tape for the morning. It combines several stretching and breathing exercises and ends with meditation. She likes it because it contains only those exercises that work best for her. Her stress management sequence is not on tape, but is a simple sequence of stretches and mental affirmations, "Take one step at a time. Don't try to do everything at once. Good, you're doing fine." This sequence is short enough for her to remember whenever she wants to relax in a stressful situation. CUE → COPE → REWARD summary: TENSE SHOULDERS → STRETCHES + AFFIRMATIONS → "GOOD, YOU'RE DOING FINE" BOOSTER

Interpersonal Stress

It is not difficult to see that most stress is interpersonal. Whether it be poor communication between lovers, excessive demands from a supervisor, inadequate feedback from a teacher, or just one of the many insults and confrontations encountered through the course of living, people create stress. In Chapters 15–20 we focus on interpersonal topics of shyness and loneliness, requests and conflict, anger, negotiation, and reaching out to others.

Chapter 15 Developing Relationships

Target Coping Skills

- Initiating, maintaining, and ending a conversation; exploring possible relationships

Purpose

- Combating loneliness and shyness
- Initiation of friendships
- Development of friendships you already have
- Coping with rejection

Example

Louis lives a lonely life. He has started college miles away from home and knows no one. He is afraid to meet others because they might reject him, or not become his friend. To deal with this general problem, Louis focused on a specific subgoal—meeting others. First he listed all the places he could meet people, including church, class, and the school cafeteria. Then he assigned himself the task of learning to "break the ice" by going to one of these places at least once a day, introducing himself to at least one person, and then treating himself to a good dinner. Once comfortable with this, he expanded his task to pursuing a conversation with at least one person a week. Here, he practiced asking questions, listening, commenting, and sharing his thoughts and feelings. This task also gave him good practice in learning to deal with his big fear, rejection. He learned to practice his people-meeting skills and to treat rejection as opportunities to grow. CUE → COPE → REWARD summary: "MEETING PLACE" → INTRODUCTION TO AT LEAST ONE PERSON → DINNER

Chapter 16 Making Requests, Saying No, and Dealing with Conflict

Target Coping Skills

Effectively stating a request, including the facts and your feelings that make your request one that should be taken seriously; outlining the benefits if your request is met, and the costs if it is not

Purpose

- Requests for raises
- Reasonable sounding requests you just do not want to honor (such as helping friends or relatives and volunteering for community organizations)
- Ask for someone else to change his or her behavior if it is hurting or offending you
- Requests in any difficult interpersonal situation

Example

Patricia wants to ask her boss for a raise. She has worked well for over three years without a single raise and feels her contributions to the company are being slighted. The moment she sees her boss, she approaches him and offers a reasonable proposal: "I have worked for this company for over three years and have not received a single raise. This frustrates me since I see others getting raises. I guess my sense of fairness tells me that good performance should be rewarded, and I feel I am performing well. I would like to put in a request for a raise this year. Frankly, getting a raise will make me feel much better about working here and going the extra mile to do a good job." After making the proposal, she praises herself for making such a good presentation. CUE → COPE → REWARD summary: CONVERSATION WITH BOSS → PROPOSAL FOR RAISE → SELF-PRAISE

Chapter 17 Dealing with Your Anger

Target Coping Skills

- Differentiating aggressive, assertive, and passive behavior
- Learning to express anger appropriately and effectively
- Learning to restrain potentially self-destructive anger
- Finding alternatives to anger

Purpose

- Response to verbal and physical attacks
- Control of impulsive anger in oneself
- Anticipation of potentially dangerous "anger" situations
- Plan for remedies when you do get out of control
- Instruction on recovery from anger

Example

James tends to "blow up" at work at the slightest provocation. Later he regrets his behavior, when it is usually too late. Using the ideas of this chapter, he learned to identify early warning signs of his anger—shaking hands and heavy breathing. Recognizing these signs gave him enough time to plan and use alternative responses that would "defuse" his anger and help solve underlying problems. Part of this involved repeating to himself the phrase, "Let's be careful. How can we solve this reasonably?" He added to his skills by learning how to "cool off" during an angry episode, and to manage anger from others. After successfully practicing, he indulged in bragging to his friends about his success. CUE → COPE → REWARD summary: SHAKING HANDS AND HEAVY BREATHING → "LET'S BE CAREFUL" REMINDER → BOAST TO FRIENDS ABOUT SUCCESS

Chapter 18 Dealing with Aggression

Target Coping Skills

- Identifying hidden aggression; managing verbal aggression

Purpose

- Response to others with hostile or manipulative behavior
- Success in making your point, or solving a problem, when others appear to be working against you
- Success in getting back on track after someone has diverted your attention through their aggression

Example

Jonah works in a secretarial pool and frequently feels under attack. Specifically, she has a problem with Delilia, one of her co-workers. Often, Delilia will display such subtly aggressive behavior as ignoring Jonah's complaints, changing the topic, and offering superficial apologies. On one occasion, Delilia initiated a rather heated and emotional argument about who is responsible for answering the phone. Using the ideas in this chapter, Jonah replied by noting Delilia's anger: "I can see this is really upsetting you." She pointed out the impact the anger was having by responding, "However, your outburst isn't solving anything. It's just upsetting people in the office." Jonah concluded with a suggestion that got to the point: "Let me suggest we put our feelings aside and try to solve this in a mature way." Later, Jonah sorted out how this was an improvement over going along with Delilia's attack. CUE → COPE → REWARD summary: DELILIA'S INITIATION OF ARGUMENT → JONAH'S RECOGNITION OF DELILIA'S ANGER → JONAH'S APPRECIATION OF IMPROVED WAY OF COPING

Chapter 19 Learning to Negotiate

Target Coping Skills

- Negotiating a solution to a conflict

Purpose

- Situations in which both parties to a conflict are willing to compromise and approach negotiation in a fair, problem-solving frame of mind
- Generation of conditions conducive to effective negotiation
- Identification of impediments to negotiation
- Tactics for deadlocked discussions

Example

Matt and Marti are working together on an important class project. However, they have serious differences on how to proceed and they decide to negotiate. First, they select a quiet and neutral setting, a picnic table in the park. They agree beforehand to think through their most important priorities. The discussion starts with Matt and Marti both stating their own positions and checking if they understand each other clearly. They then proceed with a give-and-take negotiation, with each making compromises, until a final resolution is reached. They reward themselves by going out for a drink. CUE → COPE → REWARD summary: STATEMENT OF OPENING POSITIONS → NEGOTIATION → TRIP OUT FOR A DRINK

Chapter 20 Developing Empathy

Target Coping Skills

- Listening with empathy

Purpose

- Clear understanding of what another person is thinking and feeling
- Clear and effective communication to another person of what you hear them saying
- Enhanced communication and minimized misunderstandings

Example

Claire and Charles are living together. One night Charles comes home and is clearly upset. However, he is having trouble talking about his problem. Throwing his books on the table, he blurts out, "That stupid team. Why did I even think of trying out for basketball?" Claire responds empathically, "Charles, you're really upset. Something went wrong with the team you were going to try out for today." Inside, she breathes a sigh of relief that she broke the ice and is getting to the root of the problem. Charles, feeling that Claire is clearly interested and understands, begins to talk about how he was rejected for the team he had worked so hard to join. Eventually, he talks about his feelings of frustration and anger. After about an hour, feeling a lot better, he thanks Claire, "Thanks for being here with me and letting me unload. It was really helpful." CUE → COPE → REWARD summary: ANGER TOWARDS "THAT STUPID TEAM" → EMPATHY FROM CLAIRE → RELIEF OF TENSION

Stress and Life

Coping is a life skill. Like breathing, eating, and keeping fit, it is a full-time activity. In Chapters 21–23 we take a broader look at coping and work, school, and home. We examine managing our time and priorities as a coping strategy. And we conclude with the all-important challenge of taking stock of our deficiencies, and tapping our hidden resources.

Chapter 21 Managing Work Stress

Target Coping Skills

- Identifying sources of stress at work
- Managing stress from work responsibilities
- Managing stress from amount of workload
- Managing stress resulting from work environment
- Identifying symptoms of burnout

Purpose

- On-the-job stress

Example

Rob works as a nurse in a local hospital. Although his job is difficult, he feels that much of his stress is needless. He has identified several sources of stress at the hospital: noisy, cold, foul-smelling work conditions; unclear job descriptions; and too much work. After looking at this list, it was clear that he had to talk to the supervisor and ask for help. Together, they decided to set half a day aside for a job stress workshop. In this workshop they clarified each nurse's job responsibilities. Strategies were discussed for reducing workload. Finally, they practiced giving each other helpful and constructive feedback. CUE → COPE → REWARD summary: IDENTIFICATION OF SOURCES OF STRESS → DISCUSSION WITH SUPERVISOR AND WORKSHOP → FEEDBACK AND RESOLUTION

Chapter 22 Managing Time

Target Coping Skills

- Setting goals and priorities
- Stopping "time wasters"

Purpose

- Identification of long-term and short-term priorities
- Creation of efficient weekly and daily schedules
- Effective work planning
- Solution to "feeling rushed" or "never having enough time"

Example

Gretchen never seems to have enough time to do what she wants. Even though she always seems to be busy, things just do not get done. Once she recognized how busy she felt, she decided to construct a time management plan. Using the concepts of this chapter, she carefully identified her long-term and short-term priorities. She determined one or two "absolute must" tasks for each week. After carefully monitoring how she spends her time, she discovered a number of ways in which she thoughtlessly wastes time, including vacillating between various tasks, obsessing about what should be done, and spending needless time chatting on the phone. Her reward was to schedule one extra day off that month. CUE → COPE → REWARD summary: EXCESSIVE BUSYNESS → REARRANGEMENT OF PRIORITIES AND SCHEDULE → EXTRA DAY OFF

Chapter 23 Affirming Your Resources

Target Coping Skills

- Identifying positive outcomes from a stressful situation
- Changing helplessness to optimism and resourcefulness
- Creatively generating solutions

Purpose

- Most stress situations, especially those that seem particularly difficult

Example

Francine is single and has just been laid off from a job she has held for fifteen years. She feels helpless and overwhelmed. Applying the strategies in this chapter, she first talked to a counselor to share her feelings of fear and anxiety.

In addition she tentatively began the first steps towards building a new life. Living one day at a time, she focused on simple tasks. Gradually Francine examined what general resources had been depleted through the years, and concluded that she had sunk into a rut in her job and had not developed many contacts or work-related skills. She acknowleged what resources she had, such as her ability to type, read and understand complex material, and answer the phone. Looking at the balance of her depleted and existing resources, she developed an action plan to build up her work resources. She took herself out to dinner to reward herself for this careful planning. CUE → COPE → REWARD summary: HELPLESS AND OVERWHELMED FEELING → ANALYSIS OF DEPLETED RESOURCES / IDENTIFICATION OF ACTION PLAN TO STRENGTHEN RESOURCES → DINNER

Special Problems

In the real world, even the best coping strategies can go wrong. One of the most important coping skills is dealing with special problems that can arise. In Chapters 24–28 we consider negative and interfering behaviors, relapse prevention, desensitization and stress inoculation, defense, and pain.

Chapter 24 Controlling Negative Behaviors

Target Coping Skills

- Reducing reminder cues for negative behaviors
- Reducing negative behaviors through selective punishment

Purpose

- Prevention of overeating
- Control of drinking
- Prevention of substance abuse
- Cessation of smoking
- Increase in exercise
- Any behavior that gets in the way of a reasonable coping plan

Example

Gary is seriously out of shape, and this contributes to a general lack of energy in dealing with stressful problems. He has an exercise plan, but frequently sabotages it by snacking at 4:00 P.M., the very time he should exercise. He decides on a behavior-change plan that involves punishing snacking behavior (by depriving himself of desert at dinner), and rewarding himself for exercise (by letting himself have desert). CUE → COPE → REWARD summaries: 4:00 P.M. → SNACK → PUNISHMENT OF NO DESSERT and 4:00 P.M. → EXERCISE → DESSERT

Chapter 25 Preventing Relapse

Target Coping Skills

- Identifying "high risk" stress situations in which you might fail to use a coping strategy
- Planning a "come-back" and "fall-back" coping strategy when your coping attempts do not work

Purpose

- Any potential coping failure

Example

Lisa is trying to learn to manage her time more effectively. She has learned to create a reasonable schedule, but is afraid she will resort to her old inefficient and haphazard way of getting things done. She decides to use as her relapse cue the recognition, "Oh no, I've failed my schedule." She practices a come-back strategy that involves "schedule damage control." She takes a new look at her schedule and identifies what time has been lost, and at what time it is reasonable to resume her scheduled activities. Then she takes a deep breath and reassures herself, "Fine. I'm getting practice at coming back to my schedule." CUE → COPE → REWARD summary: RECOGNITION OF FAILURE → SCHEDULE REVIEW + RESUMPTION → "FINE, I'M GETTING PRACTICE" REASSURANCE

Chapter 26 Desensitizing and Inoculating Yourself for Stress

Target Coping Skills

- Combining stress management skills to reduce stress in specific situations

Purpose

- Fears and phobias
- Anxiety in interpersonal situations
- Performance and test anxiety

Example

Violet has an intense fear of public speaking. She avoids talking in front of groups whenever possible. Applying stress inoculation training, she conditioned herself to experience public speaking with less anxiety. This involved first developing a list of ten public speaking situations, ranked from least to most stressful. Then, for each situation, she practiced imagining the initial danger cue of walking up to a podium and thinking the negative, anxiety-arousing thoughts that followed. In each practice session, she would then relax deeply so that the anxiety would go away. She then proceeded to rehearse thoughts that were more rational and useful and ended with a reward. CUE → COPE → REWARD summary: PODIUM + NEGATIVE THINKING → RELAXATION + COPING THOUGHTS → REWARD

Chapter 27 Defending Yourself When Situations Cannot Be Changed

Target Coping Skills

- Distinguishing between appropriate and inappropriate defensive strategies
- Learning what to do when everything else fails

Purpose

- Reduction of pain and discomfort of unavoidable stress
- Gain in "buying time" to figure out how to cope

Example

Reggi has just been diagnosed as having AIDS (Acquired Immune Deficiency Syndrome). He is overwhelmed with all sorts of feelings and is not sure what to do. Some days he stays home and sits in the corner. Eventually, when he finds himself sitting alone, he decides to let himself think, "Things may be OK. I'm sure they're working on a cure." Somewhat reassured, he feels less confused and helpless. He resumes work and seeks medical help. CUE → COPE → REWARD summary: SITTING ALONE → THOUGHTS THAT "THINGS MAY BE OK" → FEELINGS OF BEING REASSURED AND LESS HELPLESS

Chapter 28 Coping with Pain

Target Coping Skills

- Dealing with physical discomfort and pain

Purpose

- Acute (intense, short-term) pain
- Chronic (long-lasting) pain

Example

Ken suffers from a chronic backache. Often it prevents him from devoting full attention to his work and to his family. In attempting to deal with his pain, Ken first kept a daily diary of his pain episodes and what happened immediately before. He discovered two patterns: his backaches got worse after three hours of sitting at work, and whenever his wife would ask him to do additional work at home. Sitting at work was an easy warning sign to manage. He decided that after sitting down at work for 45 minutes, he would then stand up and walk around. Also, whenever his wife would ask him to do additional work at home, he would not passively agree. Instead, he would assertively suggest that they negotiate a reasonable division of work. Ken decided to permit himself the pleasure of a good cup of coffee each time he remembered to put his coping plans into action. CUE → COPE → REWARD summary: PERIOD OF SITTING DOWN → WALK AROUND OFFICE → COFFEE

Stressful Thinking and Worry

Is stress all in the mind? Although this idea is oversimplified, much stress is created by stressful thinking and worry. In Chapters 6–9 we will learn how to identify such thoughts, change them, stop them, and how to explore hidden thoughts and feelings that may be contributing to stress.

6

CATCHING STRESSFUL THOUGHTS

Target Coping Skills

- Identifying maladaptive, irrational thinking that contributes to needless stress

Purpose

- Stressful worry
- Most stress situations

Example

Bruce tends to make bad situations worse, but he isn't quite sure how this happens. Others have told him that thoughts can contribute to stress, but he is not aware of how his thoughts may be doing this. For a week he completes a special "thought catching" exercise that involves taking notes of what is going through his mind right after he notices he has encountered a stressful situation. When he remembers to do this, he says "good" to himself. Bruce soon discovers he creates needless stress by catastrophizing, that is, making mountains out of molehills. CUE → COPE → REWARD summary: STRESSFUL SITUATION → THOUGHT CATCHING → SAYING "GOOD" TO SELF

Here is a mystery. Imagine two people with the same problem, Thomas and Tim. Both are nurses in a local hospital who feel overworked. The problem is that their job descriptions are unclear and they end up doing more work than expected. Both have thought of a solution, that is, to talk to their supervisors about their job descriptions. However, Thomas completes this plan while Tim procrastinates and fails. Why?

The reason becomes clear when we look at how and what Thomas and Tim think when under stress. Some thoughts are conducive to stress management. For example, Thomas may have been saying to himself:

Take one step at a time.

This may make me anxious, but I can handle it.

This is a challenge, not the end of the world.

In contrast, Tim procrastinated, faltered, and failed. He may have had quite a different set of thoughts:

If I don't succeed at this, I could never live with myself. Everybody must be looking at me and thinking what a fool I am.

I've got to do this perfectly, otherwise I'm a failure.

Why do different people react differently to the same stress situation? Why do similar life events evoke such varying reactions as depression, anxiety, hostility, elation, and even indifference? The answer points to one of the most powerful and useful notions in stress management: our experience of stress is influenced by our thoughts and perceptions. In technical terms, our *cognitions* influence our reactions to stress.

We have already seen that cognitions are central to the definition of stress. We experience stress when we appraise a threat to our well-being and when we appraise coping resources to be unavailable or ineffective. It is not surprising that cognitive modification strategies are central to most approaches to stress management. Specifically, they are targeted towards changing destructive and distorted negative thoughts (Beck, Rush, Shaw, & Emery, 1979).

Psychologists have slightly differing perspectives of why negative thinking can cause stress. Some, such as Beck and Meichenbaum (1985), emphasize the harmful effect of *maladaptive* or *self-defeating* thinking. Specifically, such cognitions do not contribute to self-worth, health, or effective problem-solving. Others, such as Ellis (Ellis & Harper, 1975), emphasize the *irrational* quality of stressful cognition, that is, the extent to which it contradicts reason or the facts.

Regardless of perspective, the first step in changing stressful thinking is to identify it when it is present. To assist in this task, an impressive list of nearly 50 types of cognitive distortions have been identified (Beck, 1976; Burns, 1989; Ellis, 1977; McMullin, 1986). Those most widely applied in stress programs fall into three general categories: making inferences, evaluating how important these inferences are, and attributing responsibility or control. Knowing these types of stressful thinking can help sensitize you to your distorted thoughts.

Distortions in Making Inferences

In a sense, we are all scientists trying to figure out the problems and questions that come from living in a complex world (Kelly, 1955). The manner in which we draw conclusions, or make inferences, can contribute considerably to stress. Here are some of the most common problems people have in making inferences:

All-or-None Thinking. All-or-none thinking involves viewing the world in rigid black and white, either/or categories, and not leaving room for alternatives or shades of gray (Beck, 1976).

> Example: Matt is preparing a report for class. Although he is getting an A in the class and can afford a relatively low grade on this assignment, he still puts in extra effort. He even cancels a weekend hiking trip he had planned months ago. He thinks, "I must get an A on this paper. Any lower grade would represent failure."

Fortune-Telling. Few people can tell the future, and no one has a perfect crystal ball. And yet we engage in fortune-telling whenever we act as if we know the precise outcome of some event, precluding the possibility of the unexpected (Burns, 1980). Perhaps the most frequent form of fortune-telling is "nay-saying," which involves underrating one's coping ability or the possibility of a positive outcome. Nay-sayers assume things are always bad, they look only at the dark side and overlook the positive. They are needlessly defeatist, pessimistic, or helpless.

> Example: Geraldine has just lost her job as a clerk in a local clothing store. She liked her work, but the slow season is approaching. She thinks, "This is the last good job I'll ever have. I'll never find a job like this again."

Mind-Reading. While mind-readers in the circus might make their livings by reading minds, in everyday life attempts at "mind-reading" can be a source of needless stress. It can be dangerous to act as if we know what others want, think, or feel without asking them (McMullin, 1986).

> Example: Jose is looking for a job. He starts reading the want ads to his wife. After she criticizes the first four or five, Jose thinks, "Why does she think I don't have what it takes?"

Selective Abstraction. Those who engage in selective abstraction make up their minds too early, on the basis of little evidence (Beck, 1976). They are likely to form a conclusion based on one isolated detail of an event, ignoring other evidence.

> Example: Suzanne has just organized a party at work. Nearly everyone is having a good time. However, John is bored. Suzanne concludes, "My party is a complete failure."

Overgeneralization. Overgeneralization is similar to selective abstraction. However, instead of forming a hasty conclusion on one piece of evidence, the overgeneralizer takes conclusions already formed (regardless of the evidence) and inappropriately applies them to other situations (Beck, 1976).

> Example: Jimmie has concluded that he is "all thumbs" and cannot solve mechanical problems. His mother asks him to glue a leg back onto a table. Without thinking, he replies, "I can't do that. I'm just a mechanical dunce."

Arbitrary Inference. Most forms of distorted thinking involve leaping to conclusions. However, many people find it useful to think of it as a separate and distinct category. Here one draws inferences abritrarily in the absence of relevant evidence (Beck, 1976), and makes conclusions on the basis of the wrong facts or emotional evidence. Thinking is oversimplified.

> Example: Martin was driving to work one day and had a small accident. Another driver bumped into the rear of his car and damaged his bumper and left signal light. Although in actuality the damage was relatively slight, Martin thought: "My car is totalled. It's now a piece of junk."

Distortions in Evaluating Importance

Once you've made an inference or answered some question concerning stress, you can make things worse depending on how good, bad, or personally significant you judge things to be.

Thinking with "Shoulds," "Ought To's" and "Musts." Psychologist Albert Ellis (Ellis & Harper, 1975) in his characteristic racy style, invented the word *musturbation* to describe a special type of stressful thinking. Musturbation is a "bad habit" in which one turns wishes and desires into "shoulds," "ought to's," and "musts." Our simple wants seem to become dire necessities. In reality, few things are absolutely necessary for life to go on, although many things might well be desirable. Confusing the two can create considerable stress.

> Example: Felix is writing a report for his history class. He has typed his paper six times. It seems that every time he finishes typing, he finds a small error (a missing period or a spelling error), so he types the paper over. His thinking is, "This paper has simply got to be perfect. I can't erase or cross out errors. That's not good enough."

Awfulizing. "Awfulizers" exaggerate the importance of negative events (Ellis, 1977). They take too seriously the consequences of unmet "musts." Life has its share of frustration and disappointment, and it is healthy to recognize them. However, we awfulize when we turn simple disappointments, frustrations, and hassles into disasters. Few things merit the label "catastrophe," or "the end of the world."

> Example: Alice has been dating John every week for nearly a month. One weekend John fails to call. Alice thinks, "I feel totally depressed and worthless. Why doesn't he call?"

Awfulization is perhaps responsible for more needless stress than any other form of distorted thinking. Two variations are worth noting. *Egocentrism* involves thinking of yourself as the center of the universe. It is assuming that you have some special status, rights and privileges that others do not have (McMullin, 1986). With such imagined status, it is not surprising that the egocentric thinks life's frustrations are "just awful"; he or she is likely to complain of being unfairly victimized. *Childhood fantasy* is very similar to egocentrism. For children whose needs are easily met, love and protection are "givens." Alas, for many of them the adult world brings a rude awakening; there is no guarantee of a happy ending, or of love and wealth. Those who harbor childhood fantasies set themselves up for unpleasant and stressful surprises (McMullin, 1986).

Minimizing. We have seen that the awfulizer tends to look at the world through a stress-magnifying telescope. The minimizer can be said to look at things through the wrong end of this telescope. The significance of stress situations is understated or ignored. The importance of personal feelings, or the feelings of others, may be discounted (Burns, 1980).

> Example: Don's roommate has not returned $10 he borrowed last week. At first, Don was irritated at this apparent lack of responsibility. However, he eventually pushed the problem out of his mind, thinking, "Oh well, $10 isn't that much anyway."

Distortions in Attributing Responsibility or Control

A stress situation may well be bad. Your inferences and evaluations may be quite correct. However, how you attribute responsibility or control can make a situation even worse.

Blaming. Blaming involves inappropriately assuming that other people or circumstances are responsible for your stress (Burns, 1980; Ellis, 1977). The blamer often engages in finger-pointing, scapegoating, or idle complaining about "how bad things are."

> Example: Ben is a high school teacher frustrated by all of the low grades he gives. Although others recognize him as one of the most severe teachers in school, Ben thinks, "Why are students so poorly prepared today? They just don't have what it takes."

Personalizing. Personalizing involves pointing the finger of blame at oneself rather than at the outside world (Beck, 1976; Burns, 1980). Neutral events are seen as personal attacks. The personalizer also is likely to arbitrarily assume responsibility for a stressful situation.

> Example: Ronald is eating alone at his cafeteria at work. A group of coworkers is dining at the other end. From time to time they look in his general direction. The conversation becomes animated with lots of laughter. He thinks, "Why are they laughing at me? What's wrong with me?"

Helpless Thinking. The last form of negative thinking summarizes much of what we have been considering. Stress situations are problems to be solved. This philosophy applies to simple hassles as well as major life events. Indeed, even in situations that simply cannot be changed, it is possible to exert control over one's negative feelings through defense, relaxation, and the like. Helpless thinking is a form of giving up. It involves ignoring the coping resources most people have.

> Example: Molly was driving to the store and got a flat tire. It was relatively warm out, and cars were passing by. She just passed a service station, yet she throws her hands up in the air and cries, "Why does this have to happen now? I'm really stuck. There's no way out of this mess."

To summarize, here is a complete list of forms of negative thinking we have presented:

Distortions in Making Inferences

All-or-none thinking

Fortune-telling

Mind-reading

Selective abstraction

Overgeneralization

Arbitrary inference

Distortions in Evaluating Importance

Thinking with "shoulds, ought to's, musts"

Awfulizing (including egocentrism and childhood fantasy)

Minimizing

Distortions in Attributing Responsibility or Control

Blaming

Personalizing

Helpless thinking

You might wonder "Why are there so many kinds of negative thinking? Some seem so similar, and not all of them apply to me." It is true that some of the types of thinking we have identified overlap. For example, mind-reading is very much like arbitrary inference. However, I have decided to present a complete list as a sort of menu of ideas. Certainly, you will not select every item on the menu (I hope!). However, having many ideas to choose from makes it more likely that you will find the words that are just right in describing your type of negative thinking and how you are creating stress for yourself.

To make things simpler, when you are under stress you can look over our menu of negative thinking; however, you can achieve much the same analysis by simply asking three questions:

- What are the facts? (negative thoughts concerning inferences)
- How important is the situation really? (negative thoughts concerning evaluation of importance)
- Who's responsible—if anyone—and what can be done? (negative thoughts concerning responsibility or control)

EXERCISE 6.1 *Identifying Types of Negative Thinking*

Below are a number of brief "internal dialogues." For each, identify the type of thought distortion represented. Since many of the types of distortions we have considered overlap, there will be several answers for each:

"I would like to meet that interesting person sitting at the other side of the cafeteria. I just can't get myself to do it. She'll think I'm too forward. And I would feel just terrible."

Form(s) of negative thinking

"I just lost my car keys. I'm so stupid. How could I do such a dumb thing?"

Form(s) of negative thinking

"I know I hurt John's feelings when I didn't return his two phone calls. Oh well, things will work out."

Form(s) of negative thinking

"Listen, I've got to pass this exam or I might as well forget about ever going to college."

Form(s) of negative thinking

"Why can't I get over my depression? It's all my mother's fault. She abused me so much that I just can't get what I want."

Form(s) of negative thinking

"If you have a dream and work hard enough, nothing is impossible."

Form(s) of negative thinking

"Stress management is just silly. I can't see myself trying these stupid exercises."

Form(s) of negative thinking

"At work I've got to do everything. I can't trust anyone to do their job alone. I'm the only one I can trust."

Form(s) of negative thinking

EXERCISE 6.2 *Daily Diary*

Sometimes it is hard to know when you are engaged in negative thinking. Thoughts are fleeting things. They can speed by automatically outside of awareness. This may be the case if you answer yes to any of the following questions:

- Do you find yourself feeling physical symptoms in a stressful situation without knowing why?
- Do you find yourself feeling angry or irritated in a stressful situation without knowing why?
- Do you find yourself feeling anxious or afraid in a stressful situation without knowing why?
- Do you find yourself feeling down or depressed in a stressful situation without knowing why?
- Do you find it difficult to identify exactly what you were thinking in a stressful situation?

One useful way of catching fleeting thoughts is to complete a daily thought diary. Carry with you a few small note cards. Whenever you encounter a stressful situation, write down three things:

Cue

Negative thoughts

Costs/benefits of negative thoughts

EXERCISE 6.3 *Cartoon Captioning*

Another simple way of catching your thoughts is to draw a simple cartoon of yourself in a recent stress situation. Your cartoon doesn't have to be anything elaborate. Stick figures will do just fine. But over your head, put a "thought balloon," in which you can put the kinds of thoughts you probably had. You might also put in the kinds of thoughts others would have in a similar situation.

EXERCISE 6.4 *Talking Out Loud*

Imagine you are an actor playing out a recent stress experience. Describe your actions and speech as well as thoughts in this situation. You might imagine you are giving a running "blow-by-blow" narrative over the radio, trying to make your stress experience as lifelike as possible to listeners.

EXERCISE 6.5 *Fantasy*

Often the events of a stress situation occur so fast that they are hard to identify. You can slow them down by replaying them in your mind, by having a fantasy of what happened. In your fantasy include all the details—what you and others did, where you were, when it occurred. Include your thoughts and feelings. Imagine you are replaying a tape in your mind, one which you might have to stop and replay (like the "instant replays" on television sports) to catch hidden thoughts.

EXERCISE 6.6 *Role-Playing*

If you are in a coping team, act out a stress situation with another person acting out your part. You stand behind this person and play his or her "alter ego," that is, simply comment on what that person is thinking.

EXERCISE 6.7 *Group Brainstorming*

Many of us think similar stressful thoughts in stressful situations. It can be very useful to have a coping team brainstorm what you might have been thinking.

EXERCISE 6.8 *Labeling Your Stressful Thought*

Once you have identified what you are thinking, determine (with your coping team) what type of stressful thought it represents.

Example of stressful thought

Type of negative thinking represented

Distortions in Making Inferences

____ All-or-none thinking
____ Fortune-telling
____ Mind-reading
____ Selective abstraction
____ Overgeneralization
____ Arbitrary inference

Distortions in Evaluating Importance

____ Thinking with "shoulds, ought to's, and musts"
____ Awfulizing (including egocentrism and childhood fantasy)
____ Minimizing

Distortions in Attributing Responsibility or Control

____ Blaming
____ Personalizing
____ Helpless thinking

7

CHANGING STRESSFUL ASSUMPTIONS AND BELIEFS

Target Coping Skills

- Replacing irrational and useless thoughts with rational productive thoughts

Purpose

- Reduction of worry
- Coping with most stressful situations

Example

Ann shares a desk with another worker, Sally. Unfortunately, Sally does not put her things away and leaves a mess for Ann to tidy up. This upsets Ann considerably, but she is having a hard time confronting Sally. A number of negative thoughts get in the way, including: "I can't criticize Sally, she might think I'm too picky." In exploring this thought, Ann discovered it was part of a more general belief: "If you want people to like you, don't criticize." In her coping team, Ann carefully analyzed this belief and decided it was not rational or useful. She decided it would be much better to think, "Good friends can be frank with each other." This change of thinking was praised by her coping team. CUE → COPE → REWARD summary: NEGATIVE IRRATIONAL BELIEF → ANALYSIS OF BELIEF / REPLACEMENT WITH MORE RATIONAL AND USEFUL BELIEF → TEAM PRAISE

Stephen wants help on his math assignment. He would like to ask Kathy, but feels uncomfortable in doing so. Here is what is going through his mind:

> There's Kathy, sitting in class. I really want to ask her to help me on my assignment. I'm getting anxious. If I don't ask her, I'll feel foolish. I've got to do this perfectly, otherwise I'm a failure. Now, wait a minute. I'm blowing this out of proportion and taking this too seriously. This is a challenge, not the end of the world. This may make me anxious, but I can handle it. Gosh, everybody must be looking at me and thinking what a fool I am. Here I go again. I'm personalizing. Just focus on asking Kathy for some help. Take one step at a time. Good.

Can you see how Stephen creates stress for himself by blowing things out of proportion, personalizing, and thinking in ways that are not particularly useful or practical? Why does he do this? One reason is that Stephen harbors underlying assumptions and beliefs that are stress-producing.

Identifying Stressful Assumptions and Beliefs

Our assumptions and beliefs play a very important role in influencing how we see the world. If you assume everyone is out to get you, then you may think even the slightest comment is a hostile attack. If you think others will like you only if you "don't make waves," then you will view the slightest critical thoughts on your part as a threat to friendship.

Albert Ellis (Ellis & Harper, 1975) has developed a system of stress management and therapy called *rational emotive therapy* (RET) that focuses on how people think. To understand, let us again reconsider the preceding example of Stephen, who wanted to ask Kathy for help. Let us imagine that he is beginning to have second thoughts about his plans. His internal dialogue of worry includes:

> This is so bold, just walking up and sitting next to her. She's going to think I'm an idiot. What if she doesn't talk to me? I would feel just terrible. It would be the end of the world.

At one level, we can see a variety of troublesome thoughts. Ellis suggests that such troublesome thoughts are caused by one underlying irrational belief, in this case: "I must be loved and accepted by everyone to feel good about myself." This is clearly irrational, since it is just impossible to be liked by everyone.

Ellis has presented a system for simplifying the many negative thoughts that can contribute to stress. In fact, he summarizes the causes of stress with the letters ABC. "A" stands for an activating environmental event, such as an accident, a bad grade, or a divorce. "C" stands for your emotional and physical reactions, and your behaviors which are consequences of this event. Most people think of stress in A → C terms, that is, "My low grade made me depressed," or "My divorce is causing me to take time off from work." However, as we have seen, Ellis states that our underlying irrational thoughts, assumptions, and beliefs, the "B" in his model, are the real culprits. To illustrate:

A	**B**	**C**
Activating Event Environmental	Irrational Thoughts, Assumptions, Beliefs	Consequences (Emotional Physical, Behavioral)

It should be clear that this is the same as our 1→2→3 PROBLEM formula for viewing stress. The "activating event" is the cue that comes before stress. Emotional, physical, and behavioral consequences follow. But what about the intermediate "B," our irrational beliefs? These are the *problem* and negative thoughts that create stress.

Ellis is very well known for his list of "ten irrational beliefs." They have been debated and used by therapists and counselors for over a decade and are paraphrased below. (Can you figure out how they are irrational?)

Irrational belief #1. You must have the love and approval of everyone important in your life.

Irrational belief #2. You must prove yourself competent and adequate all the time.

Irrational belief #3. You must view life as awful, terrible, or catastrophic when things do not go your way.

Irrational belief #4. People who harm you or commit misdeeds are wicked, bad, or villainous people, and deserve severe blame, damnation, and punishment.

Irrational belief #5. If something seems dangerous or fearsome, you must become terribly preoccupied and upset about it.

Irrational belief #6. People and things should turn out better than they do. You have to view it as terrible if you do not quickly find good solutions to life's problems.

Irrational belief #7. Emotional misery comes from external pressures and you have little ability to control your negative feelings.

Irrational belief #8. You will find it easier to avoid facing life's difficulties than to undertake more rewarding forms of self-discipline.

Irrational belief #9. Your past remains all-important and, because something once strongly influenced your life, it has to keep determining your feelings and behavior.

Irrational belief #10. You can achieve happiness by inertia and inaction or by passively "enjoying yourself."

Obviously, few people go around publicly announcing such beliefs. Indeed, our stressful and irrational assumptions are often hidden, even from ourselves, and are revealed only by our thought distortions and behaviors. For example, can you tell which irrational belief the following person probably harbors?

> Clyde is a grade school teacher who suffers from chronic backaches. Although his pains have been diagnosed as stress-related, Clyde claims he is "under no stress." Each day he makes a point of arriving at school exactly one hour early to carefully clean the classroom and review notes. Everything must be just right before he can begin. When the students arrive, he passes out an exam on basic math problems. He has spent considerable time reviewing concepts the day before and expects everyone will pass. One student fails, and Clyde gets very upset, yelling, "How could you possibly fail this exam after all the work I put in?" At the end of the day, Clyde drives home. He spends the early evening washing his car, the third time this month. The slightest smudge or patch of dirt upsets him.

Clearly, Clyde believes that he must be competent or adequate all the time. This is irrational, since it is human to make mistakes. It is rewarding to excel in some things, but not everything has to be perfect. Such thinking is a sure formula for stress.

Changing Stressful Thoughts and Beliefs

Has anyone ever tried to help you by offering advice like the following?

Just think positively.

Ignore the negative and it will go away.

Repeat good thoughts to yourself and your problems will eventually disappear.

Visualize answers to your problems in your mind, and they will come to you.

Unfortunately there are many who offer such well-meaning but ineffective advice for changing thoughts and beliefs. The real job of managing stress is not so simple and requires careful, honest work. A rich assortment of techniques has been developed (Beck, et al., 1979; Burns, 1989; Ellis & Harper, 1975; Meichenbaum, 1985). We will focus on those most frequently applied, using illustrations from our friend Stephen.

Pick the Most Important Stressful Thought

When people worry, they often become preoccupied with trivial or unimportant points. From your catalog of stressful thoughts, select one that is important to you. Stress expert Burns (1989) suggests giving it a "truth score" paraphrased as follows:

5 = Absolutely true, without any doubt

4 = Probably true, with very little doubt

3 = Possibly true, with a moderate amount of doubt

2 = Possibly untrue, with some doubt

1 = Absolutely untrue, without any doubt

Recall that Stephen wanted to ask Kathy for help on a math assignment. Once again, here is his stressful thought:

> This is so bold, just walking up and sitting next to her. She's going to think I'm an idiot. What if she doesn't talk to me? I would feel just terrible. It would be the end of the world.

Stephen then evaluated his thought:

> Well, if there is one thought that really bothers me, it's that "she's going to think I'm an idiot." I really want her to approve of me. I would really take it hard if she ignored me, or simply said a few polite words and went back to her reading. If I were to give this thought a truth score, it would be a "5." It feels like it is absolutely true, without any doubt.

Evaluate and Challenge Beliefs

Take a few minutes to think about the beliefs you have identified. Ask yourself the following questions:

- What is the worst thing that could realistically happen in my stress situation?
- What facts are not consistent with my thinking?
- How is my thinking illogical?
- How does my thinking needlessly interfere with my feelings of self-worth?
- How does my thinking hamper effective problem-solving?

Here is how Stephen evaluated and challenged his stressful thinking:

> Well, let's think this through. Realistically, the worst thing that could happen when I ask for help is that she might politely refuse and return to her books. It's just not logical to assume that she will think I'm an idiot; I don't even know her. People don't generally conclude that others are idiots just because they introduce themselves, or ask for help. Furthermore, if I assume she'll think I'm an idiot, that's just going to make me more anxious and get in the way.

Construct Replacement Thoughts

Now construct replacement thoughts that are more practical and realistic. What practical and realistic beliefs do such thoughts represent? Stephen decided upon the following replacement thoughts:

> Let's be real. She may help me, she may not. There's no harm in asking. If she turns me down, I'll ask someone else.

Assess Your Original and Replacement Thoughts

Once again, use the 5-point scale to rate your original stressful thought. Rate your replacement thought. You can see how Stephen evaluated his original and replacement thoughts:

> My replacement thought seems pretty sensible. I'd give it a "4." Is she really going to think I'm an idiot? Well . . . that's unlikely. I'd rate it about a "2."

If you were working with a therapist, your work would not stop here. Additional steps include: imagining yourself in a stressful situation, then encountering and replacing stressful thoughts; practicing these situations and replacement thoughts in a "safe group" (a class or therapy group); and actually attempting to catch and replace thoughts in real-life situations.

EXERCISE 7.1 *Distorted Thinking Assessment*

Below is a list of statements that reflect some of the forms of stressful thinking considered in this chapter. Which do you display? (Check all that apply.)

____ I create stress for myself by thinking in terms of "shoulds," "musts," and "have to's."

____ I take things too seriously and fail to see them in proper perspective.

____ I tend to assume things will turn out badly even though I am not absolutely sure they will.

____ I leap to conclusions that later turn out to be a bit unrealistic.

____ I blame myself needlessly for my misfortunes.

EXERCISE 7.2 *Catching and Replacing Thoughts*

Think of a stress situation which you made worse because of what you thought. Describe the details below.

Now, analyze your situation based on the following considerations.

Catch Your Thoughts

What thoughts were you thinking with respect to this situation?

Pick the Most Important Stressful Thought

When people worry, they often become preoccupied with trivial or unimportant points. Select the most stressful thought you had. Give it a "truth rating score" from the following:

5 = Absolutely true, without any doubt

4 = Probably true, with very little doubt

3 = Possibly true, with a moderate amount of doubt

2 = Possibly untrue, with some doubt

1 = Absolutely untrue, without any doubt

____ Score for your stressful thought

Identify Cognitive Distortions and Irrational Beliefs

Next, label which types of cognitive distortion appear to be reflected by your stressful thought. If possible, identify any irrational beliefs (you may make up some if none of Ellis's ten beliefs apply).

Evaluate and Challenge Beliefs

Take a few minutes to think about the distortions and beliefs you have identified. Ask yourself the following questions:

What is the worst thing that could realistically happen in my stress situation?

What facts are not consistent with my thinking?

How is my thinking illogical?

How does my thinking needlessly interfere with my feelings of self-worth?

How does my thinking hamper effective problem-solving?

Construct Replacement Thoughts

Now construct replacement thoughts that are more practical and realistic.

Assess Your Original and Replacement Thoughts

Once again, use the 5-point scale to rate your original stressful thought. Rate your replacement thought. How true and important are they now?

____ New score for original stressful thought
____ Score for replacement thought

EXERCISE 7.3 *Costs and Payoffs*

Here is a simple way for you or your coping team to assess thoughts and beliefs. Often we persist in negative thinking because it provides certain short-term payoffs. For example, if you believe everyone will reject you, the short-term payoff for keeping to yourself is that you will not have to waste time trying to meet others. And if you believe you are helpless to improve one of your grades, then this gets you out of studying. Of course the long-term costs of these strategies are considerable—loneliness and failing school. What are the short-term payoffs and long-term costs of your stressful thoughts and beliefs?

Stressful thought or belief

Short-term payoffs	Long-term costs

Now let us examine a replacement belief that could more sensible. First, in the space provided, write a replacement thought or belief. How might it be costly in the short-term? How might it pay off in the long-term?

Replacement thought or belief

Short-term costs	Long-term payoffs

EXERCISE 7.4 *Analyzing Irrational Beliefs*

Discuss how each of Ellis's irrational beliefs are irrational and maladaptive. Then, suggest for each a replacement belief. We have completed the first example as an illustration.

Irrational belief #1. You must have the love and approval of everyone important in your life.

How it is irrational and maladaptive

It is impossible to be loved by *everyone*. It is normal and OK to be disliked by some people. Trying to win love and affection often backfires and may chase people away. The search for universal love is maladaptive.

Replacement belief

Being loved and accepted is certainly nice, but rejection is not the end of the world. Select your life goals according to what is best for *you*. When others like you, they will like the *real* you.

Irrational belief #2. You must prove yourself competent and adequate all the time.

How it is irrational and maladaptive

Replacement belief

Irrational belief #3. You must view life as awful, terrible, or catastrophic when things do not go your way.

How it is irrational and maladaptive

Replacement belief

Irrational belief #4. People who harm you or commit misdeeds are wicked, bad, or villainous people, and deserve severe blame, damnation, and punishment.

How it is irrational and maladaptive

Replacement belief

Irrational belief #5. If something seems dangerous or fearsome, you must become terribly preoccupied and upset about it.

How it is irrational and maladaptive

Replacement belief

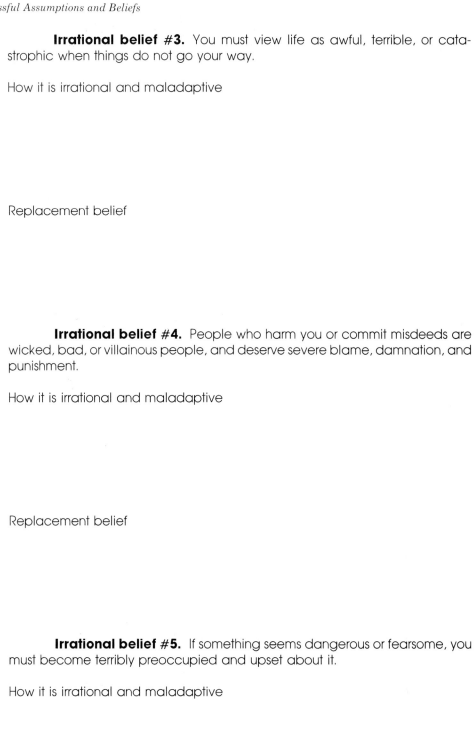

Irrational belief #6. People and things should turn out better than they do. You have to view it as terrible if you do not quickly find good solutions to life's problems.

How it is irrational and maladaptive

Replacement belief

Irrational belief #7. Emotional misery comes from external pressures and you have little ability to control your negative feelings.

How it is irrational and maladaptive

Replacement belief

Irrational belief #8. You will find it easier to avoid facing life's difficulties than to undertake more rewarding forms of self-discipline.

How it is irrational and maladaptive

Replacement belief

Irrational belief #9. Your past remains all-important and, because something once strongly influenced your life, it has to keep determining your feelings and behavior.

How it is irrational and maladaptive

Replacement belief

Irrational belief #10. You can achieve happiness by inertia and inaction or by passively "enjoying yourself."

How it is irrational and maladaptive

Replacement belief

8

REDUCING WORRY

Target Coping Skills

- Temporarily stopping needless worry

Purpose

- Supplementing techniques for reducing stressful thinking

Example

John has been trying to change his stressful thinking patterns. He is fairly good at identifying when his thoughts are needlessly stressful, and he can even think of alternatives for his stressful thoughts that are more reasonable. However, he needs a little "booster," something to help him break the pattern of obsessive negative rumination. He tries a simple exercise that involves thinking the word "STOP!" with considerable emotional intensity whenever he starts ruminating. He then does a pleasurable relaxation exercise and goes on working. CUE → COPE → REWARD summary: OBSESSIVE THINKING → THINKING "STOP!" → PLEASURABLE RELAXATION

Stressful thinking can become a persisting and annoying habit. You may well know your thinking is irrational or unproductive (if not, check Chapter 7), but you may worry anyway. Such thinking habits are called "obsessive ruminations" and fall into the same category as other minor bad habits such as nail-biting.

Why do bad habits persist? One reason is that we learn it is OK to do them in many different situations. We can see this clearly for another habit, nail-biting. You may begin biting your nails in the morning while waiting anxiously for the bus. You unconsciously reward this behavior because it keeps you from thinking about the possibility that the bus may be late. The bus stop becomes your reminder cue to start nail-biting. However, the habit extends to other cues, such as waiting for your teacher to return exams (here biting distracts you from worrying about the grade), or waiting for a date. Nail-biting has become a problem of some magnitude because it has generalized to many cues.

The same can be said for obsessive rumination. Worriers perhaps began their habit in certain, restricted circumstances, for example, worrying before exams. Worry was then rewarded. You might wonder how is worry rewarded? It always seems like such an unpleasant thing. Consider the short-term payoffs of worrying. Worrying about calling someone to make a date preoccupies you so you don't have time to make the date (you're too busy worrying). Worrying can give you a false sense of security that you are doing something productive. And, just like nail-biting, worrying extends to other cues. Soon, you are worrying before exams and while waiting for busses.

Thomas Borkovec (1985; Borkovec et al., 1983) has invented a useful little exercise for limiting worry. It is based on the idea of cutting back on the number of cues that trigger worry. The exercise is simple.

1. Closely observe your thinking during the day and learn to identify the beginnings of worry. What triggers your worry?
2. Establish a half-hour worry period to take place at the same time and in the same place every day. What is your worry period?
3. Postpone your worrying. Whenever you catch yourself worrying, put it off until your worry period.
4. Outside of your worry period, replace worrisome thoughts with focused attention on the task at hand or on anything else in your immediate environment.
5. Most important, use your daily worry period to think intensively about your current concerns.

The goal of setting up worry periods is to isolate the worry process and learn to associate it with only a limited set of circumstances.

The idea underlying worry sessions is to modify the cues linked to obsessive rumination. A different strategy, *thought stopping* (Cautela & Wisocki, 1977), focuses on modifying the consequences. As we have seen, worrying is sustained by short-term payoffs. For each additional minute of worry you can think, "Good, at least I'm doing something about this problem. I'm in control." Of course, such a pat on the back is an undeserved consequence because your worry is going nowhere. But such comforting thoughts maintain the chain of worrisome thinking.

The key to breaking a worry chain is to change the consequence. And you can do this rather simply and dramatically alone or with your coping team in three practice sessions.

You must deliberately follow your worry with a simple *aversive* consequence. You should be in a private place where you will not disturb others. Then put a bracelet-sized rubber band on one wrist.

Here is what might happen in your first session:

1. Make a list of disturbing thoughts you feel are out of your control.
   Example:
   I'm going to fail.
   Everyone is looking at me.
   People think they are better than I am.
   This is the worst thing in the world.

2. Select a target thought, one you want to eliminate.
   Example:
   I'm going to fail.
3. Discuss why you want to eliminate it. How is it self-defeating or irrational?
   Example:
   Thinking that I'm going to fail certainly doesn't help me get things done. It's irrational. How do I know for sure that I'm going to fail? That's fortune-telling. I may succeed. And if I make mistakes, I can learn from them.
4. Sit back and relax. Wait a few seconds. Start thinking your target thought. The instant you begin thinking the thought, yell the word STOP! as loud as you can and snap the rubber band. Yes, yell it out loud! This may be upsetting, but that is the point. By yelling STOP!, you break the chain.
5. Sit and wait. Relax. If the thought appears again, yell STOP! again as loud as you can while snapping the rubber band. Yell STOP! several times if necessary.

Now you are ready for your second practice session:

1. Sit back and relax. Let your mind wander. The moment you begin to think the target thought, say the word STOP! in a normal tone of voice. Snap your rubber band.
2. The next time the target thought appears, yell STOP! just like you did in the first session. Yell STOP! several times if necessary.

Your third session is even easier:

1. Sit back and relax. Once again, let your mind wander. The moment you begin to think the target thought, just *think* the word STOP! as loud as you can in your mind. Snap your rubber band. Repeat it a few times if necessary.
2. The next time the thought occurs, simply think STOP! without snapping your rubber band.

There is an additional payoff to the thought-stopping approach. Because it is impossible to think two thoughts at the same time, you simply cannot worry while thinking (or yelling) STOP!, and you help break a chain of thinking in which one worry leads to another.

EXERCISE 8.1 *Worry Session*

In this exercise, simply select your time and place for a worry session. Follow the session with a little rewarding consequence.

EXERCISE 8.2 *Thought Stopping*

Using the instructions presented in this chapter, select a thought you wish to stop. As preparation, answer the following questions:

1. List the disturbing thoughts you feel are out of your control.
2. Describe the target thought you want to eliminate.
3. Discuss why you want to eliminate it. How is it self-defeating or irrational?

After trying this technique, report to your coping team. You may even wish to do this as a group exercise with your coping team.

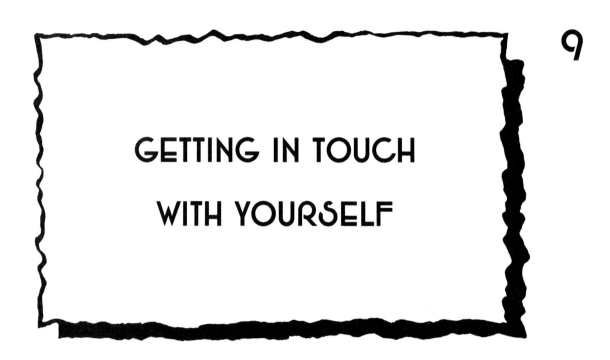

9

GETTING IN TOUCH WITH YOURSELF

Target Coping Skills

- Uncovering hidden thoughts and feelings; exploring why you are really upset, depressed, confused or anxious

Purpose

- Clarification of reasons for wanting to attempt a coping skill
- Identification of goals
- Preparation for brainstorming coping options
- Release of pent-up emotions

Example

Cynthia is starting college. Although she had planned to live on campus, financial problems are forcing her to live at home. She is alone in her room and feeling confused and "down in the dumps." Cynthia has spent hours trying to figure out why she feels so bad, but with no success. She decides to try a focusing exercise that has helped her in the past. First she sits down and makes herself comfortable. Then she lets her mind become quiet, and puts aside attempts to think about or figure out her problem. She quietly attends to her feeling of being "down in the dumps," and asks, "What is the main thing about this feeling?" Without trying to figure things out, she waits. A variety of thoughts come and go that do nothing to clarify the causes. Suddenly she has a thought that fits perfectly what she is feeling: "I don't want to live with my parents! I feel trapped! I want to live on my own!" After finishing the exercise, she treats herself with a good taco. CUE → COPE → REWARD summary: FEELING "DOWN IN THE DUMPS" → FOCUSING EXERCISE → TACO TREAT

If you take a look at the techniques presented in Chapters 6 through 8, you will notice that they all involve coping with stressful thoughts. Indeed, stress management is sometimes criticized for being too cognitive. (This can be a problem if you do not include other techniques mentioned in this book.) However, there is one technique that is both cognitive and emotional, Eugene Gendlin's (1981) *focusing*. We will present a modified version of his exercise and show how it can apply to stress management.

Clear a Space

When we are stuck with a problem, it is often because we are thinking too hard about it. We get into a mental rut trying to figure out or analyze its components. Sometimes it is better to take a break from thinking. Gendlin's exercise begins by putting aside attempts to analyze or think about a problem, and clearing a mental space.

Attend to the Gut Feeling

Often when a problem crops up, the first thing we notice is a vague feeling of discomfort. For example, you may have just finished shopping for groceries. Suddenly you stop. Something feels wrong. You may not be sure what it is, but the feeling is there. Something is wrong. Often such feelings are vague and fuzzy, such as:

"I'm a little afraid, but I don't know why."

"I feel confused. I wish I knew what was going on."

"Why am I blue and down in the dumps? I just don't know."

"I feel guilty, but I haven't done anything wrong."

"My life feels empty and incomplete. I can't put my finger on why, but that is how I feel."

These feelings can be very important. They can be the tip of an iceburg, the surface of very important underlying thoughts and emotions. The first step in uncovering what is hidden is to ask a simple question.

What Is the Gist of the Problem?

Without pushing the feeling away, analyzing it, or imposing some answer on it, simply wait. Ask yourself, "What is the gist or crux of this feeling?" And simply wait. If your mind wanders, that is OK. Then return to the question again. Remember, you are calmly attending to the *gut feeling*, not to any particular thought.

The "Zig-zag-aha" Process

As you calmly wait and attend to your gut feeling, thoughts and images will likely come and go. Again, there is nothing you have to do but wait. It is as if you were watching clouds float by in the sky, not attempting to figure them out or hold onto them. In time, a special word or image might emerge that you know in your gut perfectly fits what you are feeling. How do you know? Well, because it *feels right*.

To return to our grocery shopping example, you attend to the feeling that something is wrong, asking, "What is the gist or crux of this feeling?" Without trying to deliberately come up with an answer, you wait while attending to the feeling. The following thoughts may come up: "I haven't eaten lunch—no, that's not it . . . I spent too much—no, that doesn't feel right . . . ahh, I forgot to buy milk! Of course, that's it. That's what's wrong." Notice the "zig-zag" process in which thoughts come and are let go of until the right answer comes.

Attend to the New Gut Feeling

When a word or image comes to mind that perfectly expresses your gut feeling, a shift will occur. The feeling will open up slightly, become more clear. You will understand more of it. Here you have a choice—to repeat the process on the new gut feeling (waiting for the "crux of it"), or simply to stop the focusing exercise.

This process of uncovering feelings is hard to explain intellectually, so I will present some more examples from various students and clients.

Stephen: Feeling Blue

> Why am I so blue and down in the dumps? I've been struggling with this problem for hours. I've tried listing all my problems, ordering myself to "feel better," telling myself my negative feelings are irrational, identifying irrational goals, and nothing seems to work. Finally, I just quit. I put my thinking cap on the shelf, so to speak, and I am quietly attending to my blue feeling inside. I don't try to push it away, talk to it, or do anything. I just attend to feeling blue and ask, "What is the most important thing about this feeling?" And I wait.
>
> All sorts of mental noise come to mind. While quietly waiting, I think, "My grades aren't good enough." No, that isn't it. "I'm not working." No. "I want to watch TV tonight." No, again.
>
> I calmly wait, not trying to do a thing. Eventually it hits me. "I feel alone." That is it. That is how I really feel. My "feeling blue" is changed and now I feel both lonely and blue. I understand my feeling better.
>
> I continue with this. What is the crux, the most important thing about my "feeling blue and alone?" I again put my thinking cap aside and wait. Thoughts come and go. In time, a tear comes to my eyes as I think, "Maggie, my girlfriend. I feel so distant from her. We aren't close any more." Yes, that really hurts. That is at the core of my feeling alone and blue. And I feel a sense of relief, like a fog has lifted. I am still sad, but it is clearer, and is something I can deal with. I think about how I might get in touch with Maggie and talk about where we are going.

In this example a lot is going on. Most important, notice how the beginning gut feeling, "feeling blue," actually is at the surface of other hidden feelings such as "feeling alone, distant from Maggie." Also, notice how the initial gut feeling is often one that would be hard to deal with using problem-solving strategies. How does one get "unblue"? And notice how the hidden clarification of feeling "distant from Maggie," although painful, is at least manageable? One can begin to apply problem-solving strategies of this book.

Julia: Feeling Anxious

> I'm in class and feel anxious. What's going on? I've tried to tell myself that it is illogical to feel anxious in class, but this hasn't worked. Finally, I decided to quit trying to solve my anxiety problem and quietly attend to the feeling of tension and nervousness inside. What is the crux of this feeling? "I want to get out of class"? Well, not quite. "I want to sit next to my friend George"? No, that's not it. Ah, here it is, "I feel so intimidated looking at the professor. I feel she knows I've done something wrong."

OK, now let's keep going. No need to try to figure this new feeling out intellectually. Just attend to the feeling, "I feel so intimidated . . . I've done something wrong." Just wait and attend. Lots of irrelevant thoughts and details come to mind. Then I think of it, "I must act smart and educated whenever I talk to my professor." A silly thought, but it really fits what I feel inside. I laugh and talk to myself about the feeling. "Why must I always act smart and educated? That doesn't make any sense. I bet the professor doesn't always act smart and educated. Everyone lacks knowledge and education in something."

What is interesting in this example is how Gendlin's exercise is integrated with others presented in earlier chapters. First, an underlying thought and feeling is uncovered, "I must act smart and educated." Then, some of the cognitive techniques presented in Chapters 6 and 7 are applied in order to determine how the underlying thought is needlessly irrational and stressful. In this way, Gendlin's exercise can be a useful beginning, not only to problem solving, but to other approaches. This is illustrated in our final example.

Matt: Feeling Empty

What do I want? I've tried buying things, winning at sports, and even booze. Nothing seems to satisfy me. I feel empty and dissatisfied. Applying problem-solving techniques does not work. What are my goals? Well, that's just the problem. I don't know what I want. Once again, deep inside, I feel empty.

I put my problem-solving techniques on the shelf and quietly attend to my gut-level feeling. Yes, I can feel it in there. It is real. It's a hollow void in the pit of my stomach. I focus on this and wait, without trying to solve anything.

What is the most important, most real thing about my feeling? All my tired old answers come and go. Each feels stale. No, I don't want a new car. No, I don't want to win another game. No, I don't want a beer.

It may seem odd, but a new thought comes to mind. "I'm tired of being so self-centered. I want to give myself, to share myself with others. I'm tired of keeping it all to myself." With a sense of relief, I realize that my life has been too one-sided. I need a bit of balance. I need to learn to give and not just take.

I try to focus on this feeling of wanting to give, and nothing happens. I decide it is time to do some homework and try some goal-directed problem solving. I brainstorm various selfless goals I might consider—working at church, doing charity volunteering, helping the kids down the street with their basketball game, and so on. I then try focusing on this list, again not figuring things out. I just attend to it, and ask, "Which feels right? Which is what I really want?" My eyes center on "helping the kids down the street." It feels right. That is how I could give my time.

In this example we see problem solving and Gendlin's exercise used interchangeably. Matt starts by ceasing his problem solving. He uses Gendlin's technique as far as it will go, and then returns to problem solving. Eventually, he takes the fruits of his problem-solving efforts, a list of possible sharing activities, and applies the focusing exercise on it. Perhaps this illustrates the most important element of focusing: it is not an isolated, distinct technique, but a form of nondirective or nonanalytic "feeling through" of a problem that can be integrated with any strategy in this book.

EXERCISE 9.1 *Feeling Through a Problem*

It can be helpful to begin this exercise with 15 minutes of relaxation. (You might want to consider exercises presented in the next section.) Then, if you are in a coping team, assign one member to present the following instructions:

It is normal to feel troubled or upset from time to time. What has troubled or upset you this week? How did you feel?

[Pause 1 minute]

Now, simply attend to the feeling of being upset or troubled. There is no need to think about or figure things out. You can do this after the exercise. Just direct your attention inward and focus on the feeling, emotion, or discomfort.

[Pause 20 seconds]

Without trying to figure things out, ask yourself, "What is the gist, the most important thing about this feeling?" And simply wait. There is no need to deliberately come up with an answer. Just attend to your feeling.

[Pause 1 minute]

Thoughts may come and go. There is no need to hold onto or latch onto any single thought.

[Pause 30 seconds]

If any one thought seems special, or just right, in fitting how you feel, attend to it.

[Pause 15 seconds]

Ask yourself, "What is the gist, the most important thing about how I feel?"

[Pause 2 minutes]

And again, what are you feeling? What is the central thing, the gist?

[Pause 1 minute]

You may use the next few minutes to think about whatever you want, or to simply relax.

[Pause 1 minute]

Relaxation

Relaxation can be a powerful way of reducing potentially dangerous stress arousal, as well as preparing for and recovering from stress. Different approaches to relaxation have different effects and work for different people.

In Chapters 10–14 we will explore taking time off, physical relaxation, mental relaxation, and a variety of specialized approaches. We conclude with instructions on how to create your own relaxation program or tape.

10

TAKING TIME OFF AS A RELAXATION EXERCISE[1]

Target Coping Skills

- Learning to set time aside every day for a relaxing activity

Purpose

- General relaxation
- Preparation for physical or mental relaxation training

Example

Rosemary lives a hectic life. Not only is she an administrative assistant in a major university, but she volunteers for several charitable organizations and works for her local hospital. She wanted to do something simple to reduce

[1]Parts of this chapter were adapted by permission from Smith, J. C. (1989), *Relaxation dynamics: A cognitive-behavioral approach to relaxation*. Champaign, IL: Research Press. pp. 51–57.

tension at the end of the day. Using the ideas in this chapter, she scheduled a 30-minute period after work to read for pleasure. Rosemary was surprised how effective this simple exercise was, and congratulated herself for sticking with the schedule. Perhaps it worked because her time-off period became a "healthy habit," a sacred time that could not be touched. Perhaps it provided a useful period for self-nurturing and taking care of her own needs, rather than worrying about others. CUE → COPE → REWARD summary: END OF WORK → PLEASURE READING → CONGRATULATIONS

The most difficult problem people have when learning to relax is acquiring the habit of setting aside a daily time for relaxation. This might seem like an easy thing to do, but it is important not to underestimate the difficulties. There are many hidden forces that can get in the way. First, our society has a deep and often hidden prejudice against inactivity. Relaxation is associated with laziness and wasting time. Society tells us it is OK to take it easy *after* we have completed our work. In fact, rest and time off are just as important and meaningful as work. Second, we often have the mistaken belief that success must always be preceded by strain and toil. It can take time to see that rest-related skills are equally important.

There is a third, more insidious barrier as well. People with a high-stress pattern of living may actually become accustomed to, and perhaps even crave, a chronic high level of stress arousal. Just as the alcoholic craves alcohol when sober, the "stressoholic" craves stressful activity, even when at rest.

When you begin taking time for relaxation, you will probably experience the combined effects of society's pressures and your own addiction to stress. You may feel impatient, bored, and restless. You may want things to happen immediately. You may worry that your exercises are not working. In fact, most people quit relaxation because of these problems.

In this chapter, we are going to make relaxation easy, to help counteract the problems of stress addiction and social pressure. This exercise is relaxing in and of itself, and can serve as excellent preparation for other forms of relaxation. It is surprisingly simple: you select an easy, restful activity you already know how to do and enjoy. Then you choose a time and setting to practice your restful activity. By making your breaks easy and pleasurable, you will help overcome your resistance to relaxation. You will condition your body and mind to accept taking time off for relaxation. Once you have learned this healthy habit, you probably will begin to treat your time-off periods as special and guard them carefully for yourself.

Selecting a Relaxation Activity

First you need to select a rewarding and restful activity and then decide when to practice it. When selecting your activity, it is important to keep in mind that it should be easy for you and pleasant. For one week, try to practice it for 30 minutes every day. Remember that you will be using your relaxation to condition your body and mind to accept the discipline of setting time aside on a daily basis.

Guidelines When considering which activity to select, try to follow these guidelines:

- Select an activity that involves a minimum of movement and effort. Thus, avoid walking, jogging, sports, dancing, and similar pastimes. However, if you cannot tolerate a passive activity, an active pastime will be acceptable.

- Choose an activity that can be done alone. (Avoid talking on the phone, chatting with friends, playing games, or engaging in sex.)
- Make sure your activity is not especially goal-directed or analytic. Avoid activities that have a serious purpose, such as doing homework, practicing a musical instrument (for a class or professional purposes), solving highly complex puzzles, doing difficult reading, planning the day's activities, or working on personal problems.
- Pick an activity that is different from what you usually do. Try to think of something you find restful and enjoyable that you just have not had time to do recently. Avoid activities that you already do. For example, if you already spend time each day listening to pleasant music, do not choose this as your time-off activity.
- Choose something that is indeed fun and easy, not like a chore or burden. You should like doing it.
- Take care to select an activity that will last just about 30 minutes. It is important that you stick to this time period. If you are restless after ten minutes, continue until you have finished 30 minutes. Do not let your stress addiction get to you. If after thirty minutes you are not finished and want to continue, stop anyway. It is important that you condition your mind and body to understand that the limited period is for time off and nothing else. Consistency and discipline are very important when teaching small children, and a stress-addicted mind and body often act like cantankerous children. Be firm with both.
- Finally, avoid eating, drinking, smoking, taking drugs, and napping as relaxation activities.

Here are some time-off activities other people have chosen:

Reading

Listening to quiet music

Looking at comic books

Sewing or knitting

Solving easy puzzles

Drawing

Doodling

Playing a simple musical instrument just for fun

Daydreaming

Looking at postcards or pictures

Doing your nails

Selecting a Time-Off Period

Your next task is to pick a time to practice. As mentioned earlier, you need to practice once a day for a 30-minute session. The time you pick can have considerable impact on how successful the training is for you. You need to consider carefully what the best practice times are. Here are a few guidelines:

- Do not select a time that is within one hour after eating. During that time, blood is directed to the stomach to help digest food. As a result, you may not experience the full benefit of relaxation.

- Do not select a time when you are likely to be interrupted or distracted. For example, if your friends usually call in the early evening, it would not be a good idea to make this your time-off period.
- Do not select a time when you should be doing something else or when there is pressing unfinished business. Remember, your relaxation time is yours and yours alone. All other concerns should be put aside for the duration of the session.
- Select a time that will be relatively easy for you to keep consistent.

Selecting a Restful Setting

Where you practice your relaxation can have a considerable impact on how well it works. It is important to pick a setting conducive to physical and mental calm. The place should be dimly lit, and your relaxation chair (if you use one) should be comfortable. You also should try to minimize possible sources of distraction, such as radio, TV, ringing phones, and noisy neighbors or children. Distracting sources of discomfort (heat, noise, odors) should be eliminated as well.

You may wish to adjust your surroundings to further enhance relaxation. If you are devoting a room or corner of a room to your relaxation exercises, you might want to select a painting, sculpture, rug, or plant that is suggestive of relaxation to you. Some people find the burning of incense during relaxation particularly helpful.

Effectiveness of Time-Off Activity

Once you have tried your time-off relaxation activity, you might be interested in what science says about its potential effectiveness. There are a number of scientific studies that have compared the effectiveness of regular, informal self-relaxation (like reading, listening to music, or just sitting and daydreaming) with well known approaches such as muscle relaxation or meditation (Smith, 1989). These studies have found that for many people, regular informal relaxation is just as effective in reducing stress and tension. So something as simple as taking time off on a regular basis can be a powerful way of dealing with stress. This can be especially true for someone who lives a hectic and driven day.

However, often relaxation must go beyond casual everyday forms of rest and recuperation. What do you do when taking a break is not enough to reduce tension? In such instances, a wide range of more formal approaches are available. To these we turn in the following chapters.

EXERCISE 10.1 *Brainstorming Time-off Activities*

What restful and rewarding activities would be easy for you to do? Before making your choice, it might be helpful to brainstorm a bit. Think of as many potential relaxation activities as possible, then write them in the following space. At this time, it is not important that the activities be practical or readily possible.

Just put your critical and evaluative thinking cap aside. Let yourself be creative, and think of all the relaxation activities you might be interested in doing.

POTENTIAL TIME-OFF RELAXATION ACTIVITIES

Now, look back over this list. Think about the guidelines in this chapter. Which of the activities would be best for you? Which would you be most likely to pursue? Which would do the job of conditioning your mind and body to accept taking time off on a daily basis? Make your selection, and describe it in the space provided.

MY TIME-OFF ACTIVITY

EXERCISE 10.2 *Selecting a Time-off Period*

Here is a blank calendar for one week with half-hour time slots for each day. Spend a few minutes thinking about what your week is typically like, and then, on your calendar, reserve a 30-minute time-off period each day. On the same calendar, indicate what you would ordinarily be doing the hour before and the hour after each practice period.

MY RELAXATION SCHEDULE

TIME	SUN	MON	TUES	WED	THURS	FRI	SAT
8:00 am							
8:30							
9:00							
9:30							
10:00							
10:30							
11:00							
11:30							
12:00 pm							
12:30							
1:00							
1:30							
2:00							
2:30							

MY RELAXATION SCHEDULE (*Continued*)

TIME	SUN	MON	TUES	WED	THURS	FRI	SAT
3:00 pm							
3:30							
4:00							
4:30							
5:00							
5:30							
6:00							
6:30							
7:00							
7:30							
8:00							
8:30							
9:00							
9:30							
10:00							
10:30							
11:00							
11:30							

What is your overall assessment of your proposed schedule? Think about any problems that might arise. Now is the time to be very critical and enlist the help of your coping team. It is very easy to write a schedule, but it can be very difficult to stay with it. Here are some questions to help you evaluate your schedule:

- What interruptions might come up during your time-off period?
- How do you plan to deal with these interruptions?
- If other people are going to be around (family, roommates), what are you going to tell them so they will not interrupt you?
- What mechanical interruptions can you prevent (by disconnecting the phone, turning off TV, or closing a window)?

EXERCISE 10.3 *Evaluating Your Time-off Activity*[1]

The following words describe experiences people often have. Please carefully read each and indicate the extent to which it fits what you felt while practicing your time-off activity. Rate all the words by putting numbers in the blanks to the left. Use the following key:

[1]Adapted by permission from Smith, J. C. (1991). *Relaxation Wordlist.*

HOW WELL DOES THE WORD YOU ARE READING FIT HOW YOU FELT WHILE PRACTICING YOUR TIME-OFF ACTIVITY?

1 = Fits me not at all
2 = Fits me slightly
3 = Fits me moderately
4 = Fits me very well
5 = Fits me extremely well

____ 1. Absorbed
____ 2. Accepted
____ 3. Accepting
____ 4. Asleep
____ 5. Assured
____ 6. At ease
____ 7. Awake
____ 8. Aware
____ 9. Beautiful
____ 10. Blessed
____ 11. Calm
____ 12. Carefree
____ 13. Childlike
____ 14. Clear
____ 15. Complete
____ 16. Confident
____ 17. Contented
____ 18. Creative
____ 19. Delighted
____ 20. Detached
____ 21. Dissolving
____ 22. Distant
____ 23. Drowsy
____ 24. Energized
____ 25. Fascinated
____ 26. Floating
____ 27. Focused
____ 28. Forgetting
____ 29. Free
____ 30. Fun
____ 31. Glorious
____ 32. Glowing
____ 33. Happy
____ 34. Harmonious
____ 35. Healing
____ 36. Heavy
____ 37. Hopeful
____ 38. Indifferent
____ 39. Infinite
____ 40. Inspired
____ 41. Joyful
____ 42. Knowing
____ 43. Laid back
____ 44. Light
____ 45. Limp
____ 46. Liquid
____ 47. Loose
____ 48. Loved
____ 49. Loving
____ 50. Mysterious
____ 51. Mystical
____ 52. Optimistic
____ 53. Passive
____ 54. Patient
____ 55. Peaceful
____ 56. Playful
____ 57. Pleased
____ 58. Prayerful
____ 59. Refreshed
____ 60. Relaxed
____ 61. Rested
____ 62. Restored
____ 63. Reverent
____ 64. Selfless
____ 65. Sensuous
____ 66. Silent
____ 67. Simple
____ 68. Sinking
____ 69. Soothed
____ 70. Speechless
____ 71. Spiritual
____ 72. Spontaneous
____ 73. Strengthened
____ 74. Thankful
____ 75. Timeless
____ 76. Tingling
____ 77. Trusting
____ 78. Unafraid
____ 79. Untroubled
____ 80. Warm
____ 81. Whole
____ 82. Wonderful
____ . Total score for your time-off activity

EXERCISE 10.4 *Identifying the Effects of Your Time-off Activity*

Different approaches to relaxation have different effects. Identifying the effects of your time-off activity can help you determine if it is the best approach to relaxation for you. In the space below, list those words from the Relaxation Wordlist[1] (EXERCISE 10.3) that best fit your time-off activity.

Source: Adapted by permission from Smith, J. C. (1991a). The *Relaxation Wordlist.* Published by author, Chicago, Ill.

11

PRACTICING PHYSICAL RELAXATION TECHNIQUES

Target Coping Skills

- Three physical relaxation techniques—tensing up and letting go, stretching, and breathing

Purpose

- General relaxation
- Particular usefulness for beginners
- Reduction of physical arousal symptoms
- Stress preparation (after stress warning sign)
- Stress recovery (at consequence stage)
- Increase in general energy and alertness
- Preparation for sleep
- "Warm-up" preparation for mental relaxation exercise

Example

Jose is a basketball player. Before a game he experiences so much tension that it interferes with his game. He is particularly tense in the shoulders. In addition, his breathing is short and forced. He has found several pre-game relaxation exercises to be particularly valuable for reducing excess tension. He tightens up and shrugs his shoulders, and then lets go. Then he stretches his arms and legs out. He completes his relaxation by taking a few deep breaths. At the end, he rewards himself with a good glass of water, and begins the game. CUE → COPE → REWARD summary: PRE-GAME TENSION → RELAXATION EXERCISES → GLASS OF WATER

Physical relaxation techniques are widely used in stress clinics. They can be used, not only to prepare for and recover from stress, but also to enhance performance. They are easy to learn and produce noticeable effects rather rapidly. There are three types of physical techniques: isometric squeeze relaxation, stretching, and breathing (Smith, 1989).

Isometric Squeeze Relaxation

Isometric squeeze relaxation (also known as "progressive relaxation") is one of the most popular approaches to relaxation in the West. The most widely used variation of this approach involves tensing up and then letting go of various muscle groups, much as you might shrug your shoulders to relax. How does this approach actually create relaxation? First, many people have difficulty noticing when they are tensing up; by deliberately tightening up you can teach yourself to detect when you are tense and when you are relaxed. Also, squeezing a muscle group actually helps it to relax. It is as though you are sledding down a snow-covered hill with a slight incline, barely enough for good sledding. You might push your sled uphill a bit to get a running start. When you let go and start sliding, the extra momentum created by the uphill climb helps you to go farther. Similarly, by first tensing up a muscle group, you give it a running start, and the momentum of letting go helps you to relax.

Here are four simple steps for isometric squeeze relaxation:

1. Tighten up one muscle group while keeping the rest of the body relaxed. Do not create discomfort or pain, just a good "squeeze." Maintain the squeeze for five seconds while you attend to the sensations you have created.
2. Let go. Let your muscles go limp. If you want, you can count backwards from 30 to 1. An alternative is to count five breaths (inhalation-exhalation cycles), letting go of tension with each outgoing breath.
3. Now, simply enjoy the feelings of relaxation. Attend to how the muscle group feels. Compare the feelings of tension and relaxation.
4. Do the exercise once again before going on.

Complete instructions for each exercise are presented in the exercise section for this chapter.

Yogaform Stretching

Yoga is a very ancient and popular approach to relaxation. However, it is traditionally a mix of religion, philosophy, dietary practices, and exercises. Yogaform stretching focuses only on the physical act of stretching and unstretching. It is much slower and more passive than isometric squeeze relaxation, as you can tell from the following stretch:

> Slowly, smoothly, and gently reach your arms high up into the air. Take your time and go very smoothly, as if you were balancing a feather on each arm. Reach higher and higher until you can feel the stretch all along your arms. Then hold the stretch for about five seconds. Then, very slowly, smoothly, and gently return your arms to your lap.

Notice that, unlike isometric squeeze relaxation, yogaform stretching does not use a "tense-let go" rebound to produce relaxation. Instead, yogaform exercises actually stretch out muscle tension. It is as if each tense muscle group were a tightly coiled spring. You loosen it by gently pulling, stretching, and unstretching. Complete exercises are at the end of this chapter.

Breathing Exercises

Breathing plays an important part in both stress and relaxation. Relaxed breathing begins with the diaphragm, a drum-like muscle that separates the stomach from the abdomen. The diaphragm moves up into the chest when you breathe out, and down when you breathe in, creating the sensation of emptying and filling your abdomen with air. In addition, relaxed breathing is usually even, slow, and full.

When tense, we breathe in and out from our chests (in extreme cases, puffing our chests in and out like a boxer). The pace of breathing may be too rapid, pauses may be too short, and we may breathe too shallowly. Often breathing is uneven, rather than rhythmic.

Breathing exercises teach us to acquire more control over the breathing process and, when necessary, make greater use of the diaphragm and breath at a more relaxing pace. Some involve actively stretching, whereas others involve simply focusing on the flow of breath. For examples of breathing exercises, see the end of this chapter.

Selecting Your Exercise

Which form of physical relaxation is best for you? It is best to try each approach for a number of days. Try relaxing at different times in the day. If an exercise does not have immediate effects, try it a few more days. Then go on to a different approach. Remember that different approaches work for different people.

EXERCISE 11.1 *The Start-Off Checklist*[1]

Before beginning physical relaxation training, it is essential to make sure you are ready. Below is a relaxation "Start-Off Checklist" that covers some of the preliminaries (Smith, 1989).

- Have you selected practice times during which you are relatively unlikely to be distracted? Remember, it is not a good idea to practice when you have some other duty that has to be done.
- If you will be using a chair for your physical relaxation exercise, is it comfortable?
- Do you have a quiet place in which to practice? If you are going to practice in a place where there are other people, try to make sure you will not be interrupted. You might want to close the door to your room. Ask friends or family members not to interrupt while you are "resting." And it is OK to take the phone off the hook.
- You should not take alcohol or nonprescription drugs for at least a day before practicing. Such substances and stronger drugs (including marijuana, amphetamines, barbiturates, and psychedelic drugs) can actually make it more difficult to relax or to focus attention on what you are doing. At the very least, they can limit the extent of the effects of physical relaxation outside the session.
- You should not have a drink containing caffeine (coffee, tea, or cola) for at least two hours before practicing. Caffeine can make it more difficult to relax and to focus attention on what you are doing.

[1]Adapted with permission from Smith, J. C. (1989), *Relaxation dynamics: A cognitive-behavioral approach to relaxation.* Champaign, IL: Research Press. p. 58.

- You should not smoke tobacco for at least an hour before practicing.
- You should not eat any food for at least an hour before practicing. If you are absolutely starving, eat a carrot.
- When you are finished with your training session, come out of relaxation very slowly and gently. Arising too abruptly can be jarring and can even make you feel dizzy. Take about 60 seconds to easily open your eyes all the way. Then stretch your arms to your sides and take a deep breath.

Finally, here are some general recommendations that apply to all relaxation (Smith, 1989, pp. 23–24). Learning relaxation is like learning any other skill, whether it be swimming, driving a car, or singing: you have to start with the basics and build up; you have to practice; and you have to be patient. To ensure maximum benefit, you should practice your techniques once for 20–30 minutes a session. Moderate benefits can be obtained by practicing once a day. Less frequent practice can be useful for those who are not interested in mastering the skill of self-relaxation, but who desire a simple demonstration of specific techniques.

Do not expect immediate results, as few skills are mastered overnight. Often the effects are gradual, and different exercises will work for different people. Some exercises in this program simply may not be the right ones for you.

One important piece of advice applies to every exercise presented in this program. If an exercise makes you uncomfortable in any way, first try shortening it (doing it for 15 minutes instead of 20 to 30) and exerting less effort. If it still makes you uncomfortable, drop the exercise unless you are under professional supervision. This advice is so important that it merits repeating: if an exercise hurts, makes you dizzy, anxious or depressed, or feels unpleasant or uncomfortable in any way, ease up and spend less time at it. If the problem continues, stop the exercise, unless you are under professional supervision.

On rare occasions, relaxation exercises can have unwanted physical effects. For most people self-relaxation is comfortable and safe, but you should seek medical permission before beginning training if you now have or have had in the past any of the following conditions:

Backaches
Blackouts
Cerebrovascular accidents
Depression (severe)
Diabetes
Glaucoma
Heart disease
Hypoglycemia
Hypertension
Pregnancy (third trimester)
Thyroid disorder
Transient ischemic attacks
Any recent or serious disorder affecting bones, ligaments, or muscles

Most relaxation training manuals, including this one, warn that relaxation training can alter the required dosage levels for prescription medication, particularly for patients undergoing treatment for hypertension, diabetes, depression, anxiety, and any disorder influenced by changes in general metabolic rate. Although the potential for risk has not been consistently demonstrated, the state of relaxation itself is frequently associated with changes in general metabolic rate. As a result, need for medication may decrease (or, in a few cases, temporarily increase). If you take medication, consult with your physician before starting relaxation training.

EXERCISE 11.2 *Isometric Squeeze Relaxation Exercises*[2]

Hand Squeeze

Focus on one hand, make a fist, and let go. Repeat for other hand.

Arm squeeze

Attend to one arm, and squeeze your lower and upper right arm together, bending at the elbow. You might want to imagine that you are trying to touch your shoulder with your hand. Let go. Repeat for other arm.

Arm and Side Squeeze

Rest your hand in your lap. Press one arm to your side as if you were squeezing a sponge in the pit of your arm. Remember to keep the rest of your body relaxed. Let go. Repeat for other arm.

Back Squeeze

Attend to the back muscles that are below the shoulders. Tighten up these muscles in whatever way feels best. You might arch your back and extend your stomach and chest out. Squeeze your back muscles together, bend to one side and then the other, or even press and rub your back against the back of the chair as if you were rubbing an itch. Squeeze, and let go.

Shoulder Squeeze

Shrug the shoulders. Let go.

Back of Neck Squeeze

Gently tilt your head back. While keeping the rest of your body relaxed, gently press the back of your head against your neck. Let go.

Face Squeeze

Squeeze your jaws, tongue, lips, nose, eyes, eyebrows, and forehead all together, as if you were making a very ugly face. Let go.

Front of Neck Squeeze

Bow your head and gently press your chin down to your chest. Let go.

Stomach and Chest Squeeze

Tense your stomach and chest in whatever way feels best, by pulling your stomach in, pushing it out, or by tightening it up. Then let go.

Leg Squeeze

Attend to one leg. While keeping the rest of your body relaxed, tense the muscles by pushing your foot against the leg or back of your chair, or by pressing your legs together. Let go. Repeat for other leg.

Foot Squeeze

Curl the toes of one foot into the floor while pushing down. Let go. Repeat for other foot.

[2]Adapted with permission from Smith, J. C. (1989), *Relaxation dynamics: A cognitive-behavioral approach to relaxation*. Champaign, IL: Research Press. pp. 68–80.

EXERCISE 11.3 *Yogaform Stretching Exercises*[3]

Hand Stretch

Keep both hands resting comfortably in your lap. Slowly, smoothly, and gently open one hand. Open the fingers and easily stretch them back and apart so you can feel a good stretch (not so much that it hurts). Hold the stretch, then gently unstretch. Repeat exercise on same hand, and do it twice with left hand.

Arm Stretch

Slowly, smoothly, and gently slide one hand down your leg in front of you. Reach out and extend your arm. Do this very gracefully, as if you were balancing a feather on your hand. Reach out all the way into the air so that you can feel a good stretch all along your arm. Hold the stretch. Then slowly, smoothly, and gently unstretch. Return your arm to its resting position. Repeat with same arm and continue to other arm.

Arm and Side Stretch

Let both arms fall limply to your sides. Slowly, smoothly, and gently circle one arm and hand up and away from your body, like a slow-moving hand of a clock or wing of a bird. Imagine that you are balancing a feather on your fingertips. Extend your arm straight, and circle it higher and higher. Then circle your arm over your head so that your hand points to the other side. Stretch and arch your body as you reach and point farther and farther, like a tree arching in the wind. Hold the stretch. Then, slowly, smoothly, and gently return your arm to your side. Repeat with same arm and continue to other arm.

Back Stretch

Let your arms hang limply to each side. Slowly, smoothly, and gently relax and bow from the waist. Do not force yourself to bow. Let gravity pull your body toward your knees. It is fine to take a short breath if you need it. Feel the stretch all along the back. Hold the stretch. Then slowly, smoothly, and gently return to an upright position. Repeat.

Shoulder Stretch

Lift both arms straight out in front of you and let your fingers touch. Slowly, smoothly, and gently circle them around together, as if you were hugging a big pillow to your chest. As your hands cross, pointing in opposite directions, feel the stretch all along your shoulders. Hold the stretch. Then slowly, smoothly, and gently reverse. Return your arms to your sides. Repeat.

Back of Neck Stretch

Let your head tilt easily toward your chest. Do not force it, but simply let gravity pull your head down farther and farther. Feel the stretch in the back of your neck as you let go. Hold the stretch. Then slowly, smoothly, and gently return your head upright. Repeat.

[3]Adapted with permission from Smith, J. C. *Relaxation dynamics: A cognitive-behavioral approach to relaxation.* Champaign, IL: Research Press. pp. 88–111.

Face Stretch

Attend to the muscles of your face. Slowly, smoothly, and gently open your jaws, mouth, and eyes while lifting your eyebrows. Open wide. Feel every muscle of your face stretch. Then slowly, smoothly, and gently release the stretch. Let the tension smooth out. Let your face relax. Repeat.

Front of Neck Stretch

Now let your head tilt backward this time. Let gravity pull your head back, slowly, smoothly, and gently, just enough to feel the stretch. Do not force your head back. Let the gravity do the work for you as it pulls the heavy weight of your head. Gently and slightly open your mouth and let your head relax and fall back. Notice how the muscles in the front of the neck stretch. Hold the stretch, then gently return to your original resting position. Repeat.

Stomach and Chest Stretch

Gently lean back in your chair, arching your stomach and chest out. Feel a stretch all along your torso. Stretch your stomach and chest out more and more. Hold the stretch. Then, slowly, smoothly, and gently, release the stretch and return to your upright resting position.

Leg Stretch

Focus on one leg and slowly, smoothly, and gently stretch it out in front of you. Lift it and stretch it so that you can feel a complete stretch all along your leg. Then gently release the stretch. Slowly, smoothly, and gently let your leg return to its original resting position. Repeat and do twice with other leg.

Foot Stretch

Focus on one foot. While resting your heel on the floor (with your leg bent at knee), gently pull your toes and foot up, as if they were being pulled by strings. Let the foot and leg stretch. Feel the stretch all the way. Hold the stretch. Then slowly, smoothly, and gently unstretch. Return your foot to its original position. Repeat and do twice with other foot.

EXERCISE 11.4 *Breathing Exercises*[4]

Arm-swing Breathing

Let both arms hang by your sides. As you breathe in, circle your arms behind you very slowly, smoothly, and gently. Take in a complete breath. When you breathe out, gently and easily circle your arms around to your front and let them cross your chest as if you were hugging a pillow. Breathe in and out in a slow, relaxed pace.

Body-arch Breathing

As you inhale, gently arch back and stretch your back and let your head tilt back slightly. When you exhale, slowly and gently return to an upright position.

[4]Adapted with permission from Smith, J. C. (1989), *Relaxation dynamics: A cognitive-behavioral approach to relaxation.* Champaign, IL: Research Press. pp. 120–129.

Breathing and Bowing

Let both arms hang by your sides. As you exhale, gently and slowly bow at the waist, letting your chest and head move toward your knees. Let gravity pull you down, squeezing all the air out. When ready, slowly, smoothly, and gently sit up as you breathe in.

Bowing and Stretching

As you inhale, slowly and smoothly reach and stretch up into the air. Arch your back and gently circle both arms up toward the sky like the hands of a clock or the wings of a great bird. When you are ready to exhale, slowly circle your arms down so they hang heavily. Gently bow over, as before, letting gravity pull your body down.

Inhaling Through Nose

As you breathe in, imagine you are sniffing a very delicate flower. Let the flow of breath into your nose be as smooth and gentle as possible, so that you barely rustle a petal.

Exhaling Through Lips

Breathe out slowly through your lips, as if you were blowing at a candle flame just enough to make it flicker but not go out. Breathe in through your nose.

EXERCISE 11.5 *Evaluating Physical Relaxation with the Relaxation Wordlist*

People have different experiences to different approaches to relaxation. The Relaxation Wordlists[5] on pages 102, 103, and 104 each contain 82 words people frequently use to describe relaxation experiences. After you practice a physical relaxation activity (isometric squeeze relaxation, yogaform stretching, breathing), fill out the Relaxation Wordlist and compute your total score. Comparing this score with your score for other approaches to relaxation can help you decide which approach is best for you.

Relaxation Wordlist for Isometric Squeeze Relaxation

The following words describe experiences people often have. Please carefully read each and indicate the extent to which it fits what you felt while practicing isometric squeeze relaxation. Rate all the words by putting numbers in the blanks to the left. Use the following key:

HOW WELL DOES THE WORD YOU ARE READING FIT HOW YOU FELT WHILE PRACTICING ISOMETRIC SQUEEZE RELAXATION?

1 = Fits me not at all
2 = Fits me slightly
3 = Fits me moderately
4 = Fits me very well
5 = Fits me extremely well

[5]Adapted with permission from Smith, J. C. (1991), *Relaxation Wordlist.* Available from author.

___ 1. Absorbed
___ 2. Accepted
___ 3. Accepting
___ 4. Asleep
___ 5. Assured
___ 6. At ease
___ 7. Awake
___ 8. Aware
___ 9. Beautiful
___ 10. Blessed
___ 11. Calm
___ 12. Carefree
___ 13. Childlike
___ 14. Clear
___ 15. Complete
___ 16. Confident
___ 17. Contented
___ 18. Creative
___ 19. Delighted
___ 20. Detached
___ 21. Dissolving
___ 22. Distant
___ 23. Drowsy
___ 24. Energized
___ 25. Fascinated
___ 26. Floating
___ 27. Focused
___ 28. Forgetting
___ 29. Free
___ 30. Fun
___ 31. Glorious
___ 32. Glowing
___ 33. Happy
___ 34. Harmonious
___ 35. Healing
___ 36. Heavy
___ 37. Hopeful
___ 38. Indifferent
___ 39. Infinite
___ 40. Inspired
___ 41. Joyful
___ 42. Knowing
___ 43. Laid back
___ 44. Light
___ 45. Limp
___ 46. Liquid
___ 47. Loose
___ 48. Loved
___ 49. Loving
___ 50. Mysterious
___ 51. Mystical
___ 52. Optimistic
___ 53. Passive
___ 54. Patient
___ 55. Peaceful
___ 56. Playful
___ 57. Pleased
___ 58. Prayerful
___ 59. Refreshed
___ 60. Relaxed
___ 61. Rested
___ 62. Restored
___ 63. Reverent
___ 64. Selfless
___ 65. Sensuous
___ 66. Silent
___ 67. Simple
___ 68. Sinking
___ 69. Soothed
___ 70. Speechless
___ 71. Spiritual
___ 72. Spontaneous
___ 73. Strengthened
___ 74. Thankful
___ 75. Timeless
___ 76. Tingling
___ 77. Trusting
___ 78. Unafraid
___ 79. Untroubled
___ 80. Warm
___ 81. Whole
___ 82. Wonderful

___ Total score for isometric squeeze relaxation

Relaxation Wordlist for Yogaform Stretching

The following words describe experiences people often have. Please carefully read each and indicate the extent to which it fits what you felt while practicing yogaform stretching. Rate all the words by putting numbers in the blanks to the left. Use the following key:

HOW WELL DOES THE WORD YOU ARE READING FIT HOW YOU FELT WHILE PRACTICING YOGAFORM STRETCHING?

1 = Fits me not at all
2 = Fits me slightly
3 = Fits me moderately
4 = Fits me very well
5 = Fits me extremely well

____ 1. Absorbed
____ 2. Accepted
____ 3. Accepting
____ 4. Asleep
____ 5. Assured
____ 6. At ease
____ 7. Awake
____ 8. Aware
____ 9. Beautiful
____ 10. Blessed
____ 11. Calm
____ 12. Carefree
____ 13. Childlike
____ 14. Clear
____ 15. Complete
____ 16. Confident
____ 17. Contented
____ 18. Creative
____ 19. Delighted
____ 20. Detached
____ 21. Dissolving
____ 22. Distant
____ 23. Drowsy
____ 24. Energized
____ 25. Fascinated
____ 26. Floating
____ 27. Focused
____ 28. Forgetting
____ 29. Free
____ 30. Fun
____ 31. Glorious
____ 32. Glowing
____ 33. Happy
____ 34. Harmonious
____ 35. Healing
____ 36. Heavy
____ 37. Hopeful
____ 38. Indifferent
____ 39. Infinite
____ 40. Inspired
____ 41. Joyful
____ 42. Knowing
____ 43. Laid back
____ 44. Light
____ 45. Limp
____ 46. Liquid
____ 47. Loose
____ 48. Loved
____ 49. Loving
____ 50. Mysterious
____ 51. Mystical
____ 52. Optimistic
____ 53. Passive
____ 54. Patient
____ 55. Peaceful
____ 56. Playful
____ 57. Pleased
____ 58. Prayerful
____ 59. Refreshed
____ 60. Relaxed
____ 61. Rested
____ 62. Restored
____ 63. Reverent
____ 64. Selfless
____ 65. Sensuous
____ 66. Silent
____ 67. Simple
____ 68. Sinking
____ 69. Soothed
____ 70. Speechless
____ 71. Spiritual
____ 72. Spontaneous
____ 73. Strengthened
____ 74. Thankful
____ 75. Timeless
____ 76. Tingling
____ 77. Trusting
____ 78. Unafraid
____ 79. Untroubled
____ 80. Warm
____ 81. Whole
____ 82. Wonderful

____ Total score for yogaform stretching

Relaxation Wordlist for Breathing Relaxation Exercises

The following words describe experiences people often have. Please carefully read each and indicate the extent to which it fits what you felt while practicing breathing relaxation exercises. Rate all the words by putting numbers in the blanks to the left. Use the following key:

HOW WELL DOES THE WORD YOU ARE READING FIT HOW YOU FELT WHILE PRACTICING BREATHING RELAXATION EXERCISES?

1 = Fits me not at all
2 = Fits me slightly
3 = Fits me moderately
4 = Fits me very well
5 = Fits me extremely well

____ 1. Absorbed
____ 2. Accepted
____ 3. Accepting
____ 4. Asleep
____ 5. Assured
____ 6. At ease
____ 7. Awake
____ 8. Aware
____ 9. Beautiful
____ 10. Blessed
____ 11. Calm
____ 12. Carefree
____ 13. Childlike
____ 14. Clear
____ 15. Complete
____ 16. Confident
____ 17. Contented
____ 18. Creative
____ 19. Delighted
____ 20. Detached
____ 21. Dissolving
____ 22. Distant
____ 23. Drowsy
____ 24. Energized
____ 25. Fascinated
____ 26. Floating
____ 27. Focused
____ 28. Forgetting
____ 29. Free
____ 30. Fun
____ 31. Glorious
____ 32. Glowing
____ 33. Happy
____ 34. Harmonious
____ 35. Healing
____ 36. Heavy
____ 37. Hopeful
____ 38. Indifferent
____ 39. Infinite
____ 40. Inspired
____ 41. Joyful
____ 42. Knowing
____ 43. Laid back
____ 44. Light
____ 45. Limp
____ 46. Liquid
____ 47. Loose
____ 48. Loved
____ 49. Loving
____ 50. Mysterious
____ 51. Mystical
____ 52. Optimistic
____ 53. Passive
____ 54. Patient
____ 55. Peaceful
____ 56. Playful
____ 57. Pleased
____ 58. Prayerful
____ 59. Refreshed
____ 60. Relaxed
____ 61. Rested
____ 62. Restored
____ 63. Reverent
____ 64. Selfless
____ 65. Sensuous
____ 66. Silent
____ 67. Simple
____ 68. Sinking
____ 69. Soothed
____ 70. Speechless
____ 71. Spiritual
____ 72. Spontaneous
____ 73. Strengthened
____ 74. Thankful
____ 75. Timeless
____ 76. Tingling
____ 77. Trusting
____ 78. Unafraid
____ 79. Untroubled
____ 80. Warm
____ 81. Whole
____ 82. Wonderful

____ Total score for breathing relaxation

EXERCISE 11.6 *Identifying the Effects of Physical Relaxation*

Different approaches to relaxation have different effects. (Identifying the effects of isometric squeeze relaxation, yogaform stretching, and breathing can you determine which is the best approach to relaxation for you.) In the space below, list those words from the Relaxation Wordlist (EXERCISE 11.5) that best fit each physical relaxation exercise you tried.

Isometric Squeeze Relaxation Words

Yogaform Stretching Words

Breathing Words

12

PRACTICING MENTAL RELAXATION

Target Coping Skills

- Thematic imagery, fantasizing, visualizing
- Meditating

Purpose

- General relaxation
- Alleviation of worry
- Self-exploration
- Reduction of physical arousal symptoms
- Stress preparation (after stress warning sign)
- Stress recovery (at consequence stage)
- Increased general energy and alertness
- Preparation for sleep

Example

Beth has tried physical relaxation techniques without success. She finds them frustrating and a bit boring. She does like to relax by engaging in a pleasant fantasy, or going off by herself to a quiet place. Recently she learned imagery and meditation in a stress management class, and seems to like what these techniques offer. Even before breakfast, she takes a 20-minute fantasy/relaxation break. Breakfast becomes a pleasant reward. CUE → COPE → REWARD summary: WAKING UP → FANTASY/RELAXATION → BREAKFAST

Many people relax simply by thinking relaxing thoughts. Put simply, this is the idea underlying two forms of mental relaxation, thematic imagery and meditation.

Thematic Imagery

Thematic imagery is an approach most people know something about. Have you ever simply sat back and let your mind wander in a peaceful daydream? That is thematic imagery (Smith, 1989, 1990, 1991). Specifically, you select a relaxing theme and then dwell on it. Your theme should be passive, simple, and relaxing (resting on a meadow rather than playing football). Involve most of your senses—what you see, hear, feel against your skin, and smell.

The five general themes of imagery involve travel, outdoors/nature, water, indoor settings, and wise person/healing forces. Following are specific examples of each (Smith, 1991, 1992):

- Travel Imagery (going by train, airplane, hot air balloon or floating through the air or outer space)
- Nature/Outdoor Imagery (being on a grassy plain, nature trail, mountain top or hill, in the woods or a garden)
- Water Imagery (being on the beach, in a boat, in a small pond, tub or pool, walking in the mist or rain, or going fishing)
- Indoor Imagery (relaxing on a bed or sofa, in a winter cabin, a vacation dream house, a church or temple, or childhood home)
- Wise Person/Healing Forces (finding comfort in Buddha, Jesus, a wise rabbi, priest or nun, a therapist; the energy of the sun, cleansing water, energizing air.)

Once you select your theme, introduce the details, as if you were creating a painting or motion picture. For example, if your theme is *Standing on a Mountain Top*, you might include the following details:

What You See

Distant clouds

Far-away trees

The valley below

Birds above

Patches of flowers

A solitary deer

What You Hear

Rushing water of a stream

Mountain wind

A lonely bird

Silence

What You Feel Touching Your Skin

Heat of the sun

A cool breeze

Spray of water

Soft moss

A cool rock

What You Smell

Mountain air

Flowers

Fragant trees

Practicing thematic imagery is very simple. Close your eyes and involve all your senses. You might want to check the wordlist at the end of this chapter for some relaxation phrases or affirmations to "spice up" your imagery.

Meditation

People often confuse meditation with imagery, but they are quite different. Meditation is perhaps the simplest and most difficult of relaxation exercises. When most people first try meditation, they often try to do too much. The instructions are really very simple (Smith, 1987):

Calmly attend to a simple stimulus
Gently return your attention after every distraction
Again and again and again

Many people have some idea of what meditation is like without learning a specific meditation technique. Here is one experience that may seem familiar.

> I am outdoors admiring the clouds. My mind is free from worry and distraction. I have no urge to analyze the clouds. I simply attend, calmly and peacefully attend, as they lazily float by . . .

Meditation begins with a simple stimulus, the clouds for example. The stimulus should be so simple that it does not evoke distracting thoughts and feelings. Thus, try not to meditate on the thematic imagery themes we have just discussed. They are just too complex.

When you meditate, your mind will wander. You will start thinking about things other than your meditation stimulus, noticing outside noises, and worrying about what you are doing. It is important to remember that it is OK to be distracted while meditating (Smith, 1989). Meditation is not a concentration exercise. The goal is not to glue your attention to your stimulus as if you were playing a video game. Let yourself be distracted. After every distraction calmly return your attention to your stimulus. Meditation is not so much a concentration exercise as it is an exercise in returning attention after every distraction, an exercise in "coming home."

When you meditate, you might want to think of what happens when you take a pet for a walk on a path through the woods. The pet may innocently wander from the path again and again. Each time the pet wanders, you gently and lovingly return him without making a big thing of it. You realize that eventually your pet will learn to stay on the path, and that each wandering gives you a chance to reinforce the returning motion again. Similarly, each time you return your attention to your meditative stimulus, you gently condition your mind to attend for longer periods of time. Once again, it is OK to be distracted. It is only through being distracted that you have the opportunity to practice returning your attention and to build your meditative skills.

There are at least six basic meditations I like to teach (Smith, 1987, 1992). Since different meditations work for different people, it is a good idea to find what works best for you. Here are the instructions:

Rocking Meditation. Rocking meditation is a very simple technique rarely taught in the Western world. However, I have found it to be one of the most effective and satisfying forms of meditation because it is very soothing. Whether you are sitting in a rocking chair or in a boat in a pond, or even rocking a child in your arms, the gentle back-and-forth motion can be very peaceful. In rocking meditation, begin by rocking back and forth in your chair. When you are comfortable with this, make your rocking movements increasingly smaller and gentler so that someone watching you would not notice that you are rocking at all. Gently attend to your rocking motion, and after every distraction gently return your attention . . . again and again and again.

Breathing Meditation. Breathing is basic to most forms of relaxation. Breathing meditation simply involves letting the word "ONE" float through your mind every time you passively and effortlessly exhale. It is important not to force the word "ONE" or try to make it go at a particular speed or volume. Simply wait for it to float through your mind, almost as if you were attending to clouds floating by in the sky.

Meditation on a Relaxing Word. The most widely practiced form of meditation in the Western world involves focusing on a simple relaxing word or syllable. You can use the words "calm" or "peace," or simply pick a soothing syllable like "Hmmm" or "Ommm." Simply let your word or syllable float through your mind, again like clouds. Let it go in its own way, speed, and volume. All you have to do is attend, and return your attention every time your mind wanders.

Meditation on a Visual Image. This meditation involves attending to a visual mental image with your eyes closed. First, pick a very simple, unchanging mental image. You might use a star, pebble, dewdrop, candle flame, or religious symbol. Avoid complex images such as those used in thematic imagery. These can stir up distracting thoughts and associations. Calmly attend to your image, and return your attention after every distraction.

Meditation on an External Visual Stimulus. This meditation is a bit different. Begin by opening your eyes half way, almost as if you were half asleep. Then select a very simple and unchanging external object, like a doorknob, light, or candle. Easily gaze on this object. Whenever your mind wanders, gently return to the stimulus.

Meditation on Sounds. Here is another meditation on external stimuli. This time, quietly attend to the coming and going of everything you hear around you. There is no need to dwell on any particular sound or to try to figure sounds out. Simply wait for a sound, acknowledge what you hear, let go, and continue attending. You might think of this in a way similar to watching bubbles that gently float by on a stream, or clouds that float by in the sky. Of course, you cannot hold onto or keep bubbles or clouds. Simply watch them come and go. Attend, let go, and attend again.

EXERCISE 12.1 *Thematic Imagery Worksheet*

Indicate here the theme you have selected for your imagery exercise:

List all the relaxing things you see:

List all the relaxing things you hear:

List all the relaxing things you feel touching your skin:

What relaxing fragrances do you smell?

EXERCISE 12.2 *Meditation Worksheet*

Select which meditation you want to practice.

Rocking meditation.

Breathing meditation.

Meditation on a relaxing word. (What is your word?)

Meditation on a visual image. (What is your image?)

Meditation on an external visual stimulus. (What is the stimulus?)

Meditation on sounds.

EXERCISE 12.4 *Evaluating Mental Relaxation with the Relaxation Wordlist*

People have different experiences to different approaches to relaxation. The Relaxation Wordlists on pages 111 and 112 contain 82 words people frequently use to describe relaxation experiences. After you practice thematic imagery or meditation, fill out the Relaxation Wordlist[1] and compute your total score. Comparing this score with your score for other approaches to relaxation can help you decide which approach is best for you.

[1]Adapted by permission from Smith, J. C. (1991). *Relaxation Wordlist.*

Relaxation Wordlist for Thematic Imagery

The following words describe experiences people often have. Please carefully read each and indicate the extent to which it fits what you felt while practicing thematic imagery. Rate all the words by putting numbers in the blanks to the left. Use the following key:

HOW WELL DOES THE WORD YOU ARE READING FIT HOW YOU FELT WHILE PRACTICING THEMATIC IMAGERY?

1 = Fits me not at all
2 = Fits me slightly
3 = Fits me moderately
4 = Fits me very well
5 = Fits me extremely well

____ 1. Absorbed
____ 2. Accepted
____ 3. Accepting
____ 4. Asleep
____ 5. Assured
____ 6. At ease
____ 7. Awake
____ 8. Aware
____ 9. Beautiful
____ 10. Blessed
____ 11. Calm
____ 12. Carefree
____ 13. Childlike
____ 14. Clear
____ 15. Complete
____ 16. Confident
____ 17. Contented
____ 18. Creative
____ 19. Delighted
____ 20. Detached
____ 21. Dissolving
____ 22. Distant
____ 23. Drowsy
____ 24. Energized
____ 25. Fascinated
____ 26. Floating
____ 27. Focused
____ 28. Forgetting
____ 29. Free
____ 30. Fun
____ 31. Glorious
____ 32. Glowing
____ 33. Happy
____ 34. Harmonious
____ 35. Healing
____ 36. Heavy
____ 37. Hopeful
____ 38. Indifferent
____ 39. Infinite
____ 40. Inspired
____ 41. Joyful
____ 42. Knowing
____ 43. Laid back
____ 44. Light
____ 45. Limp
____ 46. Liquid
____ 47. Loose
____ 48. Loved
____ 49. Loving
____ 50. Mysterious
____ 51. Mystical
____ 52. Optimistic
____ 53. Passive
____ 54. Patient
____ 55. Peaceful
____ 56. Playful
____ 57. Pleased
____ 58. Prayerful
____ 59. Refreshed
____ 60. Relaxed
____ 61. Rested
____ 62. Restored
____ 63. Reverent
____ 64. Selfless
____ 65. Sensuous
____ 66. Silent
____ 67. Simple
____ 68. Sinking
____ 69. Soothed
____ 70. Speechless
____ 71. Spiritual
____ 72. Spontaneous
____ 73. Strengthened
____ 74. Thankful
____ 75. Timeless
____ 76. Tingling
____ 77. Trusting
____ 78. Unafraid
____ 79. Untroubled
____ 80. Warm
____ 81. Whole
____ 82. Wonderful

____ Total score for Thematic imagery

Relaxation Wordlist for Meditation

The following words describe experiences people often have. Please carefully read each and indicate the extent to which it fits what you felt while practicing meditation. Rate all the words by putting numbers in the blanks to the left. Use the following key:

HOW WELL DOES THE WORD YOU ARE READING FIT HOW YOU FELT WHILE PRACTICING MEDITATION?

1 = Fits me not at all
2 = Fits me slightly
3 = Fits me moderately
4 = Fits me very well
5 = Fits me extremely well

___ 1. Absorbed	___ 29. Free	___ 57. Pleased
___ 2. Accepted	___ 30. Fun	___ 58. Prayerful
___ 3. Accepting	___ 31. Glorious	___ 59. Refreshed
___ 4. Asleep	___ 32. Glowing	___ 60. Relaxed
___ 5. Assured	___ 33. Happy	___ 61. Rested
___ 6. At ease	___ 34. Harmonious	___ 62. Restored
___ 7. Awake	___ 35. Healing	___ 63. Reverent
___ 8. Aware	___ 36. Heavy	___ 64. Selfless
___ 9. Beautiful	___ 37. Hopeful	___ 65. Sensuous
___ 10. Blessed	___ 38. Indifferent	___ 66. Silent
___ 11. Calm	___ 39. Infinite	___ 67. Simple
___ 12. Carefree	___ 40. Inspired	___ 68. Sinking
___ 13. Childlike	___ 41. Joyful	___ 69. Soothed
___ 14. Clear	___ 42. Knowing	___ 70. Speechless
___ 15. Complete	___ 43. Laid back	___ 71. Spiritual
___ 16. Confident	___ 44. Light	___ 72. Spontaneous
___ 17. Contented	___ 45. Limp	___ 73. Strengthened
___ 18. Creative	___ 46. Liquid	___ 74. Thankful
___ 19. Delighted	___ 47. Loose	___ 75. Timeless
___ 20. Detached	___ 48. Loved	___ 76. Tingling
___ 21. Dissolving	___ 49. Loving	___ 77. Trusting
___ 22. Distant	___ 50. Mysterious	___ 78. Unafraid
___ 23. Drowsy	___ 51. Mystical	___ 79. Untroubled
___ 24. Energized	___ 52. Optimistic	___ 80. Warm
___ 25. Fascinated	___ 53. Passive	___ 81. Whole
___ 26. Floating	___ 54. Patient	___ 82. Wonderful
___ 27. Focused	___ 55. Peaceful	
___ 28. Forgetting	___ 56. Playful	___ . Total score for Meditation

EXERCISE 12.5 *Identifying the Effects of Mental Relaxation*

Different approaches to relaxation have different effects. Identifying the effects of thematic imagery or meditation can help you determine if either is a good approach to relaxation for you. In the space below, list those words from the Relaxation Wordlist (EXERCISE 12.4) that best fit your thematic imagery or meditation.

Thematic Imagery Words

Meditation Words

13

USING SPECIALIZED RELAXATION STRATEGIES

Target Coping Skills

- Practicing self-suggestion to relax
- Shortening relaxation

Purpose

- Development of brief relaxation strategies for special situations
- Detection of relaxing activities in everyday life
- Overcoming difficulties in learning to relax

Example

Bill is having some trouble learning relaxation. When he tries a technique, he gets distracted and finds it hard to continue, yet he wants very much to enhance his ability to relax. In this lesson he learned three useful tools. First, he identified everyday activities he already does that are forms of relaxation. He discovered that he can become deeply relaxed after 30 minutes of jogging, so he carefully schedules a jogging session at 5:00 P.M. every other day. After jogging, he indulges in a good shower. In addition, he sought the assistance of a health professional to learn the use of special biofeedback equipment to help him determine when he is most tense and most relaxed. Finally, he learned some very brief relaxation exercises that can be practiced on the bus or at work. CUE → COPE → REWARD summary: 5:00 P.M. → JOGGING → A GOOD SHOWER

Understanding Relaxation More Deeply

To understand the goals of specialized approaches to relaxation, it is important to understand relaxation itself more deeply. As we have seen, relaxation can first help reduce unhealthy and unproductive levels of tension. To elaborate, each of us has a built-in stress energy "fight or flight" response. As we have seen earlier, our bodies can automatically prepare for vigorous, emergency action. Our heart pumps hard. We breathe more rapidly. Muscles become tense. In all, hundreds of changes take place as the adrenalin flows. The stress energy response is absolutely essential for survival. It provides a football player with that needed shot of energy to make a touchdown, and gives a youngster the energy to run from a neighborhood dog. However, this fight or flight response can also be triggered by events that are not life-threatening, such as worry, everyday hassles, and even the alarm clock. The result is that many of us experience unhealthy levels of stress, a problem that can contribute to a variety of illnesses, as well as reduced work productivity and ability to enjoy life.

Often deep relaxation can help counter excessive levels of stress energy. However, such relaxation is not achieved through watching television, reading books, or drinking a beer. Some strategies that are especially effective are everyday relaxation, mini-relaxation and biofeedback. Skill at deep relaxation can enable one to evoke a healthful and restorative "relaxation response," a pattern including reduced heart rate, breathing rate, and muscle tension that is the opposite of the stress response.

Relaxation training is not over once you have mastered the relaxation response. This goal is only the beginning. Central to all relaxation is the acquisition of three basic mental skills—*focusing*, *letting be*, and *openness*, as depicted in the following examples:

> It was a very hectic day. Everything was happening at once. Dogs were barking, the phone was ringing, sirens were going off and children were playing noisily outside. I decided I needed to relax and drove a few miles to the local beach. There, everything was quiet. I could simply attend to one thing, the waves and nothing else. It was very relaxing.
>
> School was making me very tense. I had hundreds of things to do. At first I started reading a chapter in my English text, then I started working on my paper. I switched to answering letters until I opened my Biology text. Finally, I decided to make my life a bit simpler and easier and do one thing at a time. I picked up my English book. I worked on it for a good hour and put everything else aside.
>
> It was a rough day and I needed to relax, so I filled my tub with hot water and simply settled into it. After a few minutes, I started to really relax. My body started to feel as though it was melting. Tension seemed to melt away. I never had this feeling before and at first it upset me. I almost got out of the tub until I decided that my melting sensations were a normal part of relaxation. I let myself enjoy them.

The person in the first example who thinks, "I'm going to attend to one thing . . ." has, in a simple way, decided to focus or to quietly attend to a restricted stimulus. In the second example, the statement, "Do one thing at a time" represents a decision to let go of unnecessary striving and take a stance of "letting be" toward the world. Finally, the student who realizes that his sensations of melting in the tub are just a sign of normal relaxation has learned to be more open and to tolerate new experiences.

We can now define relaxation skills more formally. *Focusing* is the ability to attend to a simple stimulus for an extended period of time; *letting be* describes the ability to stop excessive goal-directed and analytic activity; and *openness* is the ability to tolerate and accept experiences that may be uncertain, unfamiliar, or paradoxical. These basic skills are what make all relaxation work, from isometric squeeze to meditation. Indeed, they are essential to all effective and rewarding activity. The singer must, above all, focus on his or her performance—not the crowd or yesterday's problems. The student must be able to attend to the simple task of studying and display a stance of "letting be" concerning other distracting chores that might be tackled. The scientist must be open to the new and unexpected.

Practitioners of yoga, zen, prayer, or muscle relaxation are essentially doing the same thing—honing and refining their ability to focus, letting other distracting tasks "be," and accepting experiences that may be uncertain, unfamiliar, and paradoxical. A person is deeply relaxed when he or she has truly learned to focus and maintain a stance of letting be and openness.

But to be deeply effective, relaxation must go beyond the skills we have discussed. Deep relaxation often requires a rethinking of personal philosophies, those lasting thoughts people have about what is real, important, and worthy of action. For example, if you firmly believe that the most important thing in life is to be liked by everyone, it is easy to see how you might have trouble relaxing. Your craving to be liked and accepted could easily create considerable distracting tension. Here are some other philosophies that can get in the way of relaxation (Smith, 1991):

"I am not capable of making my life better."

"Things will automatically get better on their own."

"I do not feel good about myself when I am less than totally successful at work or school."

"Unless others love and accept me, I can't feel at peace with myself."

To learn to relax, you will eventually need to change such tension-creating beliefs. Developing personal philosophies more conducive to relaxation is perhaps the most challenging task. Some of these philosophies include (Smith, 1991):

"My selfish worries are distractions that fog awareness of a deeper reality."

"The meaning of life becomes more apparent to me in the quiet of relaxation."

"Live one day at a time."

"First things first."

"My urgent concerns seem less important when seen in broader perspective."

"There are more important things than my everyday hassles."

"At the deepest level I can feel at peace with myself—I am an OK person."

"God's will be done."

Everyday Relaxation

One way of enhancing relaxation is to look for everyday activities that enhance focusing, passivity, and receptivity as well as your relaxation philosophies. You can use the following relaxation wordlist (introduced in previous chapters) to evaluate the activities that come to mind. These are 82 words I have found to be most associated with focusing, passivity, receptivity, and relaxation philosophies. Here is the list:

Absorbed	Knowing
Accepted	Laid back
Accepting	Light
Asleep	Limp
Assured	Liquid
At ease	Loose
Awake	Loved
Aware	Loving
Beautiful	Mysterious
Blessed	Mystical
Calm	Optimistic
Carefree	Passive
Childlike	Patient
Clear	Peaceful
Complete	Playful
Confident	Pleased
Contented	Prayerful
Creative	Refreshed
Delighted	Relaxed
Detached	Rested
Dissolving	Restored
Distant	Reverent
Drowsy	Selfless
Energized	Sensuous
Fascinated	Silent
Floating	Simple
Focused	Sinking
Forgetting	Soothed
Free	Speechless
Fun	Spiritual
Glorious	Spontaneous
Glowing	Strengthened
Happy	Thankful
Harmonious	Timeless
Healing	Tingling
Heavy	Trusting
Hopeful	Unafraid
Indifferent	Untroubled
Infinite	Warm
Inspired	Whole
Joyful	Wonderful

Source: Adapted by permission from Smith, J. C. (1991a). *The Relaxation Wordlist*. Published by Author, Chicago, IL.

Can you think of everyday activities most likely to evoke feelings described by these words? Perhaps when you take an early morning walk you feel "peaceful," "calm," and "aware." Maybe taking a shower makes you feel "soothed" and "tingling." One very useful relaxation skill is to recognize everyday activities that enhance relaxation, and schedule these activities on a regular basis.

Biofeedback

Here is an experiment you might want to try. First find your pulse. You can do this by gently resting your thumb on one of the large blood vessels in your wrist or neck. For 30 seconds count your heart rate and record it here:

Now take five minutes to relax. Immerse yourself in a relaxing fantasy or daydream. Let go and really get into it. Then take your heart rate again. What is your ending heart rate?

If you have a thermometer, tape it to the center of your palm. Make sure the silvery bulb sensor is touching your palm. Wait about a minute and record your temperature.

And now, for about five minutes, imagine your hand is in soothing, warm water. Let the phrase, "My hand is warm and heavy, warm and heavy" gently float through your mind like an echo. There is no need to force your hand to feel anything. Then read your temperature again.

If you are doing this exercise with a coping team, compare notes. About half of you will note a reduced heart rate after relaxing and an increased hand temperature following the suggested phrase. These are normal physiological signs of the relaxation response.

This exercise also demonstrates a useful relaxation tool called *biofeedback*. Biofeedback involves using sensing equipment to "read" how tense or relaxed your body is. The thermometer is a biofeedback device. A doctor's stethoscope is a biofeedback device for measuring heart rate. Biofeedback equipment is available for measuring a number of physiological tension and relaxation indicators, including:

Physiological activity	**Measure**
Heart beat	Electrocardiogram (EKG)
Perspiration; emotional sweating	Electrodermal activity (EDA)
Electrical activity of the brain	Electroencephalogram (EEG)
Stomach contractions	Electrogastrogram (EGG)
Muscle tension and activity	Electromyogram (EMG)
Eye movement	Electrooculogram (EOG)
Volume of blood flow at a peripheral site; respiration	Plethysmograph
Blood flow	Temperature
Pressure	Blood pressure

Many people tune out feelings of tension that are chronic. We often tune out chronic sources of discomfort, such as street noises and the sounds of air conditioners. Biofeedback devices can let us know when we are tense, and what parts of our bodies might be most in need of relaxation.

In addition, biofeedback can give us a quick sign of when relaxation is working. Just as we saw in our two experiments, taking physiological readings can let us know immediately if a technique is working. If your heart rate went down and your temperature rose, then you know the exercises you tried were working. If these measures did not change, then the exercises were not working.

Somatic Focusing[1]

Biofeedback equipment is used by health professionals to test out a wide range of relaxation exercises. However, many begin with some easy *somatic focusing* or *autogenic* exercises. Such exercises are particularly well suited for biofeed-

[1]Adapted by permission from Smith, J. C. (1989). *Relaxation dynamics: A cognitive-behavioral approach to relaxation*. Champaign, IL: Research Press. pp. 134–136.

back, since they target biological processes. They are also easy for beginners since they reflect everyday relaxation sensations many of us already recognize. For instance, how does your body feel after a hot bath or massage? What kinds of thoughts and images go through your mind? Maybe you feel warm and heavy, or your breathing might seem cool and refreshing. You might even picture a warm beach or a refreshing breeze. Such experiences are normal and usually reflect that physical, or somatic, relaxation is taking place.

When you are tense, the blood vessels in your fingers constrict. This results in the cold, clammy hands many experience under stress. However, when you relax, these same blood vessels dilate or expand. Blood flow to the extremities increases, and you feel warm. Similarly, when your muscles relax, you are more likely to feel their weight. (Have you ever been so relaxed that you felt that you simply could not get up?) There are many physical sensations that signify that relaxation is taking place. It is possible to create and enhance relaxation by doing nothing more than thinking thoughts related to such somatic relaxation processes. This is a strategy frequently used in hypnosis, autogenic training (Luthe, 1965), Kundalini yoga (Rama, Ballentine, & Ajaya 1976), and some forms of Zen meditation (Kapleau, 1965). It is the idea underlying somatic focusing.

In somatic focusing, simply let images and words float through your mind that suggest *physical* relaxation feelings. Common phrases include (Smith, 1989):

- My hands are warm and heavy, warm and heavy.
- My hands and arms are tingling and relaxed, tingling and relaxed.
- My breathing is slow and easy, slow and easy.
- My heartbeat is easy and rhythmic, easy and rhythmic.
- My stomach is cool and soothed, cool and soothed.
- My forehead is cool and peaceful, cool and peaceful.

A wide range of mental images can be used to enhance these physical sensations, including:

- Warm water, air, or sand
- Fingers gently massaging your skin
- Cool air or water gently touching your skin
- Sunlight penetrating and warming your muscles

The point is not to force relaxation, but to passively let words and images float through your mind while you remain indifferent concerning what actually happens. It is as if you were repeating a meaningless nursery rhyme, or watching clouds float by in the sky. Such an attitude of indifference is important in order to help the suggestions actually work. Here is an exercise that can demonstrate the difference between active and passive thinking (Smith, 1989):

> First, let your right hand drop to your side. Then, actively and effortfully try to make your hand feel warm and heavy. Work at it. Exert as much effort as you can trying to actively and deliberately will your hand to feel warm and heavy.
>
> Now simply relax. Let your hand fall limply by your side. Without trying to accomplish anything, simply let the phrase "My hand is warm and heavy" repeat in your mind. Let the words repeat on their own, like an

echo. All you have to do is quietly observe the repeating words. Do not try to achieve warmth and heaviness. Just quietly let the words go over and over in your mind. While thinking the words "warm and heavy," you might want to imagine your hand in warm sand, or in the sun, or in a warm bath. Pick an image that feels comfortable, and simply dwell on it.

The first task illustrates active thinking, the second passive thinking. Most people find that passive thinking is more effective at fostering somatic focusing relaxation.

Mini-relaxation Finally, if you already practice a form of relaxation, it is possible to create a short version to practice in special places, for example, at work, on the bus, or while waiting in line. Such *mini-relaxation* can be very useful for extending relaxation into everyday life. There are three ways of making a mini-relaxation:

1. Take one part of a relaxation exercise you already practice. Use this as your mini-relaxation. For example, if you practice yoga for 30 minutes every day, you probably stretch several parts of the body such as the arms, legs, or back. Take one stretch, say a leg stretch, and make it your mini-relaxation.
2. Whenever you practice your complete relaxation sequence, end it by breathing out deeply and thinking the word "calm." After doing this for several weeks, the simple act of breathing out while thinking "calm" can be enough to evoke some relaxation. This then becomes your mini-relaxation.
3. Whenever you practice your complete relaxation sequence, end it by quietly repeating to yourself a soothing affirmation that conveys the deeper meaning of relaxation to you. You might repeat:

"One day at a time."

"First things first."

"I'm an OK person."

"God's will be done."

The repetition of this phrase in the course of a busy day can serve as your mini-relaxation to reduce stress.

EXERCISE 13.1 *Evaluating Your Everyday Activities with the Relaxation Wordlist*

People have different experiences to different approaches to relaxation. The Relaxation Wordlist on the following page contains 82 words people frequently use to describe relaxation experiences. After you engage in an everyday activity that you think might be relaxing, fill out the Relaxation Wordlist and compute your total score. Comparing this score with your score for other approaches to relaxation can help you decide which approach is best for you.

First, name the everyday activity you think might be relaxing:

Relaxation Wordlist for Everyday Relaxation Activity

The following words describe experiences people often have. Please carefully read each and indicate the extent to which it fits what you felt while engaged in the following everyday activity: ______________________. Rate all the words by putting numbers in the boxes to the left. Use the following key:

HOW WELL DOES THE WORD YOU ARE READING FIT
HOW YOU FELT WHILE ENGAGED IN AN EVERYDAY ACTIVITY YOU FIND RELAXING?

1 = Fits me not at all
2 = Fits me slightly
3 = Fits me moderately
4 = Fits me very well
5 = Fits me extremely well

____ 1. Absorbed
____ 2. Accepted
____ 3. Accepting
____ 4. Asleep
____ 5. Assured
____ 6. At ease
____ 7. Awake
____ 8. Aware
____ 9. Beautiful
____ 10. Blessed
____ 11. Calm
____ 12. Carefree
____ 13. Childlike
____ 14. Clear
____ 15. Complete
____ 16. Confident
____ 17. Contented
____ 18. Creative
____ 19. Delighted
____ 20. Detached
____ 21. Dissolving
____ 22. Distant
____ 23. Drowsy
____ 24. Energized
____ 25. Fascinated
____ 26. Floating
____ 27. Focused
____ 28. Forgetting
____ 29. Free
____ 30. Fun
____ 31. Glorious
____ 32. Glowing
____ 33. Happy
____ 34. Harmonious
____ 35. Healing
____ 36. Heavy
____ 37. Hopeful
____ 38. Indifferent
____ 39. Infinite
____ 40. Inspired
____ 41. Joyful
____ 42. Knowing
____ 43. Laid back
____ 44. Light
____ 45. Limp
____ 46. Liquid
____ 47. Loose
____ 48. Loved
____ 49. Loving
____ 50. Mysterious
____ 51. Mystical
____ 52. Optimistic
____ 53. Passive
____ 54. Patient
____ 55. Peaceful
____ 56. Playful
____ 57. Pleased
____ 58. Prayerful
____ 59. Refreshed
____ 60. Relaxed
____ 61. Rested
____ 62. Restored
____ 63. Reverent
____ 64. Selfless
____ 65. Sensuous
____ 66. Silent
____ 67. Simple
____ 68. Sinking
____ 69. Soothed
____ 70. Speechless
____ 71. Spiritual
____ 72. Spontaneous
____ 73. Strengthened
____ 74. Thankful
____ 75. Timeless
____ 76. Tingling
____ 77. Trusting
____ 78. Unafraid
____ 79. Untroubled
____ 80. Warm
____ 81. Whole
____ 82. Wonderful

____ Total score for Everyday Relaxation Activity

EXERCISE 13.2 *Identifying the Effects of an Everyday Relaxation Activity*

Different approaches to relaxation have different effects. Identifying the effects of your everyday relaxation activity can help you determine if it is the best approach to relaxation for you. In the space below, list those words from the Relaxation Wordlist (EXERCISE 13.1) that best fit your everyday relaxation activity.

EXERCISE 13.3 *Selecting a Mini-Relaxation*

List the relaxation exercises you now do.

Select one portion of an exercise from this list that you could use as a mini-relaxation.

What word or affirmation can you say after your relaxation exercise to use as a mini-relaxation?

14

MAKING A RELAXATION SCRIPT OR TAPE

Target Coping Skills

- Combining favorite relaxation exercises for a specific relaxation goal
- Making a relaxation tape

Purpose

- Advanced relaxation for those who have already mastered more than one relaxation technique
- Any relaxation goal, including managing stress, combating insomnia, waking up refreshed in the morning, enhancing creativity and productivity, enhancing personal growth and exploration

Example

Sheila has spent many years exploring the relaxation marketplace. She has tried yoga, self-hypnosis, meditation, and a variety of relaxation tapes. However, none seem just right for her relaxation goals. She wants a brief exercise to use whenever her shoulders begin to feel tense, an early-warning stress cue. Using the exercises in this chapter, she made her own relaxation tape for the morning. It combines several stretching and breathing exercises and ends with meditation. She likes it because it contains only those exercises that work best for her. Her stress management sequence is not on tape, but is a simple sequence of stretches and mental affirmations, "Take one step at a time. Don't try to do everything at once. Good, you're doing fine." This sequence is short enough for her to remember whenever she wants to relax in a stressful situation. CUE → COPE → REWARD summary: TENSE SHOULDERS →

TABLE 14-1 Summary of Steps for Writing a Relaxation Script

Selection of Script Components
1. Relaxation goal
2. Unifying idea
3. Specific exercises
4. Sequence of exercises

Elaboration of Components
1. Incorporation of unifying idea
2. Imagery details
3. Deepening words and affirmations
4. Sequence coherence

Refinement of Components
1. Anticipation of setbacks
2. Relaxation reinforcements
3. Pauses and silences
4. Termination segment

STRETCHES + AFFIRMATIONS → "GOOD, YOU'RE DOING FINE" BOOSTER

After you have tried many types of relaxation, how do you know what is right for you? Over the years, I have found that often the best answer is to combine the techniques that have worked for you into your own unique relaxation sequence. If you want, you can read this sequence into a tape recorder to make your own relaxation tape. Since script writing involves making many revisions, I recommend using a word processor.

There are many payoffs from making your own relaxation script:

- You include only what works for you. (Different exercises work for different people.)
- You can select exercises that facilitate your relaxation goal. (Different exercises can be better for different goals.)
- Since you are inventing your own relaxation format, you are more likely to take it seriously and to practice it regularly.
- You can include special suggestions and exercises to deepen your relaxation.
- Finally, you can use your relaxation as a reminder of personal philosophies you find conducive to living a life of peace and calm.

Here are the three basic steps for making a relaxation script and tape:[1] First you select the basic components of your relaxation sequence. Then you return and add elaborations and refinements to each basic component. We will explain each step, and illustrate how one person, Sue, developed her script. We conclude with some sample scripts others have written.

Selection of Script Components

Relaxation Goal First you must decide why you want to relax. Some possible goals include: managing stress, healing, combating insomnia, relaxing at the end of the day, waking up refreshed in the morning, enhancing creativity and productivity,

[1]Adapted by permission from Smith, J. C. "The basic protocol: Rules for making a relaxation script" in *Cognitive-behavioral relaxation training: A new system of strategies for treatment and assessment*. Copyright 1990, Springer Publishing Company, Inc., New York 10012, pp. 102–134.

and self-exploration and growth. Sue selected as her goal, "daily relaxation for self-expression and growth."

WHAT IS YOUR RELAXATION GOAL?

Unifying Idea

A relaxation exercise sequence acquires structure and meaning from a unifying idea, a statement of what it is all about. Once a unifying idea is selected, it should be woven into exercise components (we will learn how to do this later). There are five possible types of unifying ideas:

- *Exercise rationale.* Often a unifying idea is little more than a statement of the process you think makes relaxation work. For example, you may believe relaxation is effective for reducing stress because it triggers a "relaxation response," or that it enhances creativity because it "taps your unconscious."
- *Exercise goal.* A relaxation goal can be simply the reason for adopting the exercise, for example, combating insomnia, waking up refreshed for the day, preparing for work, or communing with nature.
- *Affirmation of personal philosophy.* Unifying ideas can be affirmations of personal relaxation philosophies, for example, "Live in the present moment," "God's will be done," "Let go of that which cannot be changed," or "Trust the powers within you."
- *Relaxation metaphor or image.* Metaphors or symbolic images of relaxation can be unifying ideas. The theme of *peaceful woods* might encompass many types of exercises. For example, a gentle breeze could symbolize breathing exercises; trees slowly bowing in the wind, stretching exercises; and the silence of approaching evening there, a meditation. Note how these images are not only peaceful in their own right, but are suggestive of specific relaxation exercises. To take an example we will use again later, the theme of *waves crashing on the shore* can involve a variety of exercises. The energy that builds and releases with each crashing wave can suggest shrugging the shoulders and letting go, as well as taking in a deep relaxing breath and exhaling tension. The dissolving of each wave into the sand can be linked with mental images suggesting "heaviness, tingling, and dissolving tension." And the quiet wind that flows across the water before the next wave can suggest relaxed breathing.
- *Relaxation story.* A unifying idea can be something of a very simple story, providing all elements are linked to the relaxation exercises, increasing relaxation, and ending in deeper relaxation. For example, the theme of waves crashing on the shore just mentioned is a bit of a story: a wave builds up, crashes, dissolves into the sand, and a quiet wind blows.

It is important to put your unifying idea in your own words. You can also use a favorite poem, prayer, piece of literature, or lyrics of a song as your unifying idea. Returning to our model script-writer, Sue has selected the image of sitting on the banks of a mountain stream as her unifying idea.

WHAT IS YOUR UNIFYING IDEA?

Specific Exercises

Next, select which relaxation exercises you want to include in your sequence. You can pick as few or as many as you want. If you are including mental imagery or fantasy, pick a theme that reflects your unifying idea. Be sure to write down the detailed instructions for each exercise.

Sue has selected yoga stretching, breathing, imagery, and meditation as her preferred approaches:

Back stretch (bow over and touch the ground; reach up and touch the sky)

Deep breathing and breathing out through lips

Imagery

Meditation

WHAT SPECIFIC RELAXATION EXERCISES DO YOU WANT TO INCLUDE?

Sequence of Exercises

The next step is to decide an exercise practice order consistent with your unifying idea. It is generally best to proceed from active and complex exercises to those that are passive and simple, although variations from this pattern can be effective. It is possible to combine exercises, for example, a hand and arm stretch, or hand squeeze and hand stretch. We are now ready to examine excerpts from Sue's script. Detailed instructions for yoga and breathing are presented, although those for imagery have been left for later.

SUE'S SCRIPT: EXERCISE SELECTION AND SEQUENCE

[Yoga stretch]

Sit up slowly, smoothly, and gently. Reach and stretch higher and higher into the sky, as if you were touching the clouds. Reach all the way. And then pause. Then, slowly, smoothly, and gently return to an upright, seated position.

[Breathing]

Take in a deep breath, filling your lungs completely.
Gently exhale.
Let the air flow out of your lips with every breath.

[Imagery: Sitting on the banks of a mountain stream. To be added later]

[Meditation]

WRITE DOWN THE EXPLICIT INSTRUCTIONS FOR EACH EXERCISE IN THE ORDER YOU WISH.

Elaboration of Components

Incorporation of Your Unifying Idea

Each exercise you have selected should be linked with your unifying idea. For example, in the following segment the unifying idea is "breathing out tension and settling into calm." Notice how this idea is woven into each exercise:

Take in a deep breath. Slowly bow over, let go, and exhale.

Let tension begin to melt and flow out with your breath.

Now you become more calm. While sitting upright, breathe in deeply and slowly and exhale. As you begin to settle into calm, let more and more tension dissolve and float away.

Now, let yourself become even more calm. Let your breathing be effortless and unforced. Simply attend to each incoming and outgoing breath. Let yourself settle into a deeper and deeper state of relaxation as any remaining tension begins to flow away.

As we noted earlier, a unifying idea can also be expressed in a simple story, for example, "a leaf floating down the river," "a bubble rising to the surface of the pond," or "the sun dissolving a block of ice into a puddle of water." Here is an example in which such story changes are woven into a sequence of exercises:

Tense and let go. Imagine a bubble is released from the floor of a pond.

Quietly attend to your breathing. Let tension flow with every outgoing breath. As breath flows, the bubble slowly rises.

In your mind's eye simply attend to the bubble as it reaches the surface. It touches the air and bursts, releasing its tension. Let go of remaining feelings of tension.

Here are some more examples of how to weave a unifying idea into your sequence:

Unifying idea: The relaxation goal of preparing for sleep.

Tense up your shoulders. Let go. Release some of the tension that keeps you from sinking deeper into a pleasant drowsy state.

Take in a deep breath. Let the air soothe you and calm your tensions. Let the air out, and sink into sleepiness.

Quietly breathe in and out. With each outgoing breath, let yourself become more quiet and drowsy.

Unifying idea: A personal relaxation philosophy, "Let go of needless control."

Tense up your shoulders. Notice how this is like trying to control your life. Now relax and let go. Let go of the needless tension you have created.

Take in a deep breath. Hold it in, like you hold in needless tension through the day. Then relax and breathe out, letting go of needless tension.

Unifying idea: The image of a ball of string unwinding.

Tense up your shoulder muscles. Imagine tension as a tight ball of string. Then relax and let go. Imagine the ball of string slowly unwinding.

Take in a deep breath. Hold it in. Then relax and breathe out. The ball of string unwinds even more.

Unifying idea: A palm tree bowing in the wind.

Imagine you are a palm tree bowing gently in the wind.

You are on a very peaceful island, far away from any cares and concerns.

The wind blows, and subsides.

As the wind begins to blow, gently stretch.

Stretch farther and farther, feeling a good complete stretch.

And as the wind subsides, gently unstretch, releasing your tension.

Here again is Sue's script. Note how her unifying idea, the image of sitting on the banks of a mountain stream, is repeated in each exercise.

SUE'S SCRIPT: UNIFYING IDEA

[Yoga stretch]

Imagine you are sitting on the banks of a mountain stream. You bow over, gently touching the water. Let tension dissolve into the water.

Sit up slowly, smoothly, and gently. Reach and stretch higher and higher into the sky, as if you were touching the clouds. Reach all the way. And then pause. Then, slowly, smoothly, and gently return to an upright, seated position.

[Breathing]

Take in a deep breath, filling your lungs completely.
Gently exhale.
Let the air flow out of your lips with every breath.
The only sound you hear is the quiet flow of breath and a quiet mountain stream.

[Imagery: Sitting on the banks of a mountain stream]

[Meditation]

NOW ADD SUGGESTIONS OF YOUR UNIFYING IDEA. ADD ONE SUGGESTION NO MORE THAN ONCE EVERY FOUR SENTENCES.

Imagery Details

If you selected imagery, visualization, fantasy, or daydream to be a part of your script, now is the time to elaborate and add details. The same is true if you want a meditation. Select your meditation focus. Once again, make your details tie in with your unifying idea. We will now take a look just at Sue's imagery and meditation exercises.

SUE'S SCRIPT: IMAGERY AND MEDITATION ELABORATIONS

[Imagery: Sitting on the banks of a mountain stream]

Now, quietly attend only to the image of sitting on the banks of a cool, refreshing mountain stream.
Your feet gently swing in the cool, refreshing water.
Tension flows down each leg, into your toes, and is dissolved and carried away by the water.
You can see the clear, sparkling water, smell its clean spray, and feel the warm sun on your skin.
Attend with all of your senses to this beautiful, relaxing moment.

[Meditation]

Quietly attend to the coming and going of the present moment.

INCLUDE IMAGERY AND MEDITATION ELABORATIONS. SEE CHAPTER 11 FOR ADDITIONAL ADVICE.

Deepening Words and Affirmations

An exercise sequence can be enhanced by "spicing it up" with words that suggest relaxation. You can choose from the same relaxation wordlist we have introduced elsewhere:

Absorbed	Knowing
Accepted	Laid back
Accepting	Light
Asleep	Limp
Assured	Liquid
At ease	Loose

Awake
Aware
Beautiful
Blessed
Calm
Carefree
Childlike
Clear
Complete
Confident
Contented
Creative
Delighted
Detached
Dissolving
Distant
Drowsy
Energized
Fascinated
Floating
Focused
Forgetting
Free
Fun
Glorious
Glowing
Happy
Harmonious
Healing
Heavy
Hopeful
Indifferent
Infinite
Inspired
Joyful
Loved
Loving
Mysterious
Mystical
Optimistic
Passive
Patient
Peaceful
Playful
Pleased
Prayerful
Refreshed
Relaxed
Rested
Restored
Reverent
Selfless
Sensuous
Silent
Simple
Sinking
Soothed
Speechless
Spiritual
Spontaneous
Strengthened
Thankful
Timeless
Tingling
Trusting
Unafraid
Untroubled
Warm
Whole
Wonderful

Source: Adapted from Smith, J. C. (1991a) *The Relaxation Wordlist.* Chicago, IL: Available from Author.

In addition to using these words individually as relaxation "seasonings," you can incorporate them into special deepening phrases. These should be introduced no more than once every four sentences. Some examples might include:

Let your fingers become *warmer* and *warmer.*

Let your body feel *lighter* and *lighter.*

You are becoming more *centered.*

You are feeling more and more *aware.*

Let yourself feel more *calm* and *loose.*

You can also add phrases that affirm your own thoughts and philosophies concerning the deeper side of relaxation. These should be introduced no more than once every ten sentences. Here are some examples.

My selfish worries are distractions that fog awareness of a deeper reality.

God loves me and has a plan for my life.

The meaning of life becomes more apparent to me in the quiet of relaxation.

My urgent concerns seem less important when seen in broader perspective.

There are more important things than my everyday hassles.

At the deepest level I can feel at peace with myself—I am an OK person.

I choose to live one day at a time and not worry about things that cannot be changed.

I choose to quit creating unnecessary pain and tension for myself by ignoring my true feelings.

God's will be done.

If a poem, passage of literature, prayer, or lyrics of a song express what relaxation means to you, by all means try to weave it into your script.

We can now return to Sue. She has selected the phrases "become more and more still," "sink more and more deeply into a pleasant state of relaxation," "your mind becomes peacefully centered," and "time is like a river, each crisis passes and is forgotten." Note how these, plus such phrases as, "Let the tension dissolve . . . let tension dissolve" enhance relaxation.

SUE'S SCRIPT: PHRASES SUGGESTING THE DEEPENING OF RELAXATION

[Yoga stretch]

Imagine you are sitting on the banks of a mountain stream. You bow over, gently touching the water. Let tension dissolve into the water.

Sit up slowly, smoothly, and gently. Reach and stretch higher and higher into the sky, as if you were touching the clouds. Reach all the way. And then pause. Then, slowly, smoothly, and gently return to an upright, seated position.

Sink more and more deeply into a pleasant state of relaxation.

[Breathing]

Take in a deep breath, filling your lungs completely.
Gently exhale.
Become more and more still.
Let the air flow out of your lips with every breath.
The only sound you hear is the quiet flow of breath and a quiet mountain stream.

[Imagery: Sitting on the banks of a mountain stream]

Now, quietly attend only to the image of sitting on the banks of a cool, refreshing mountain stream.
Become more and more still.
Your feet gently swing in the cool, refreshing water.
Tension flows down each leg, into your toes, and is dissolved and carried away by the water.
You can see the clear, sparkling water, smell its clean spray, and feel the warm sun on your skin.
Your mind becomes peacefully centered.
Time is like a river, each crisis passes and is forgotten.
Attend with all of your senses to this beautiful, relaxing moment.

[Meditation]

Quietly attend to the coming and going of the present moment.

INSERT WORDS AND PHRASES TO DEEPEN RELAXATION

Sequence Coherence

An exercise sequence that is just a random chain of calisthenics is uninteresting and easily forgotten. A number of strategies can enhance the coherence of a sequence, the degree to which separate parts fit together.

If your relaxation sequence includes several general approaches (yoga, breathing and meditation, for example), elements of one approach can be *integrated* into others. For example, breathing exercises can be separately featured in a relaxation sequence or woven into "tense-let go" or yoga stretching:

Take a deep breath as you tighten up the muscles.

Hold the muscles tighter and tighter.

As you let go, gently exhale.

Slowly, smoothly, and gently stretch.

Stretch farther and farther.

Gently take in a deep breath as you stretch completely.

Very slowly, smoothly, and gently release the stretch while exhaling.

Similarly, if you like imagery and fantasy, specific images can be integrated into other physical exercises to weave them together:

As you let go of your tension, imagine a tight ball of string slowly unwinding. Bit by bit, each string relaxes as you let go of tension more and more completely. Gently and easily the entire wad becomes more and more loose.

As you stretch, imagine you are a tree. Your arms are the branches gracefully bending in the wind. With every breeze, you bend, and release your tensions.

You are by the seashore. As each wave approaches the shore, you take a deep breath. As the wave splashes against the shore, you gently exhale and release your tensions.

An exercise can be used to *frame* a sequence. Here, an element that appears at the start of a sequence can be repeated at the end. The end version may be modified to reflect deepened relaxation. For example, a set of exercises might begin with the image of an unsettled pond, its wind-blown surface symbolizing distraction and unnecessary effortful striving. An appropriate ending could be a still, quiet pond. Similarly, you might begin and end a sequence with a deep breathing exercise. The initial exercise might be performed with some vigor and effort whereas the final version would be conducted with greater calm.

The skilled use of *metaphor* can interrelate and summarize components of an exercise and provide subtle transitions between exercises. For example, initially a yoga sequence might be described as similar to a tree bending in a wind. Later on, actual stretching instructions might be replaced with a summarizing metaphor; you stretch to the instructions, "You are a tree bending in the wind, bending slowly, smoothly, and gently." Eventually, the same metaphor can serve as a cue for a mental imagery sequence, "Imagine a tree bending." When metaphors are woven into an exercise sequence, they can serve not only as a unifying and transitional device, but as a recurring cue or reminder that the exercise sequence is growing deeper.

Returning to Sue, we can see that she has modified her script by introducing repeated instructions for "exhaling through the lips" to help add unity to her sequence.

SUE'S SCRIPT: COHERENCE

[Yoga stretch]

Imagine you are sitting on the banks of a mountain stream. You bow over, gently touching the water. Let tension dissolve into the water.

Sit up slowly, smoothly, and gently. Reach and stretch higher and higher into the sky, as if you were touching the clouds. Reach all the way. And then pause. Then, slowly, smoothly, and gently return to an upright, seated position.

Sink more and more deeply into a pleasant state of relaxation.
Quietly open your lips and let tension flow with every breath.
Let the flow of breath be as gentle as the flow of a quiet mountain stream.

[Breathing]

Take in a deep breath, filling your lungs completely.
Gently exhale.
Become more and more still.
Let the air flow out of your lips with every breath.
The only sound you hear is the quiet flow of breath and a quiet mountain stream.
Let your flow of breath be as gentle as a mountain stream.

[Imagery: Sitting on the banks of a mountain stream]

Now, quietly attend only to the image of sitting on the banks of a cool, refreshing mountain stream.
Become more and more still.
Your feet gently swing in the cool, refreshing water.
Tension flows down each leg, into your toes, and is dissolved and carried away by the water.
Quietly open your lips and let tension flow with every breath.
The flow of breath is as gentle as a mountain stream.
With every outgoing breath, let go of your worries over the past and future.
You can see the clear, sparkling water, smell its clean spray, and feel the warm sun on your skin.
Your mind becomes peacefully centered.
Time is like a river, each crisis passes and is forgotten.
Attend with all of your senses to this beautiful, relaxing moment.

[Meditation]

Quietly attend to the coming and going of the present moment.

ADD WORDS SUGGESTING COHERENCE

Refinement of Components

Anticipation of Setbacks

You are now about finished with your script. In relaxation, setbacks are common: attention wanders, expected relaxation effects do not occur, unexpected experiences are encountered, one forgets to practice, negative thoughts interfere with relaxation, and coping failures in everyday life increase tension. It is useful to expect such setbacks and deal with them through special phrases introduced in your script. For example, you might tell yourself, "Distractions are normal and can indicate that relaxation is uncovering hidden stresses. Relaxation is like any other skill, it takes time to work. Sometimes deeper levels of relaxation can create unexpected feelings and sensations." Here are some more examples:

Whenever you notice you are thinking about something unrelated to relaxation, picture yourself letting go of this thought as if it were a butterfly you are holding and releasing.

Give each distracting thought to your relaxation as if you were giving a gift.

Say to yourself, "What an interesting distraction. OK, back to my relaxation."

Say to the distraction, "Thank you," and return to your exercise.

Imagine dropping each distraction into a deep space as though you were dropping pebbles into a pond.

Let distracting thoughts and pictures stay in your mind if they want. But they stay in the background while you return to your exercise.

Imagine each distraction to be a form of stress release that enables you to relax better.

ADD ANTICIPATIONS OF SETBACK TO YOUR SCRIPT

Relaxation Reinforcements

One way of deepening and strengthening relaxation is to introduce a few words of encouragement and support and to highlight pleasurable, rewarding aspects of relaxation. Such reinforcements can be presented as direct statements ("Very good") or as phrases combined with other instructions ("It is good to let go of the cares of the day.") Some reinforcing phrases include:

There is no need to push yourself, you are doing fine.

Move at a pace that feels comfortable to you.

Notice the pleasant feelings you have created.

It is OK to let yourself sink deeper into relaxation.

When you let go and attend to relaxation, you are doing well. Take care not to introduce reinforcements for thoughts that may not be present. For example, the reinforcement, "It is good that you are completely relaxed" may actually create needless worry and tension if you are not, in fact, completely relaxed. It is better to reinforce relaxation attempts ("It is good to begin to put aside the cares of the day") as well as the general direction of relaxation ("It is good to become more focused.")

It is important to withhold reinforcements from thoughts not conducive to relaxation. For example, it is OK to *experience* distractions during a session, but pursuing them for any length of time reinforces the tendency to become distracted. Also, by reacting to a distraction by feeling disturbed or upset, one appraises the distraction as major and important. It is better to treat distractions as passing and insignificant.

Sue's reinforcements are tied into her affirmation of a relaxing philosophy: "In this silent moment, you realize that all things come and go. It is good. You are doing fine. It is a time of deep inner peace and joy."

ADD YOUR REINFORCING PHRASES TO YOUR SCRIPT

Pauses and Silences A relaxation sequence should include frequent pauses and periods of silence. It is at moments when nothing is being said or done that the effects of an exercise can begin to take hold. There are also times during an exercise when you might want to be left in silence, for example, during meditation. Finally, beginning script writers tend to be too stingy with pauses; it is better to write in too many than too few.

Termination Segment A relaxation sequence should not end abruptly. Gently state that the relaxation sequence is now over. Gradually return to the outside world and end with a good stretch or deep breath. A termination segment can include a suggestion that the pleasant feelings of relaxation will carry over to the rest of the day.

We are now ready to take a look at Sue's completed script, including her anticipation of setbacks, reinforcing segments, pauses, and a termination segment:

SUE'S COMPLETED SCRIPT

[Yoga stretch]

Imagine you are sitting on the banks of a mountain stream. You bow over, gently touching the water. Let tension dissolve into the water.

[Pause]

Sit up slowly, smoothly, and gently. Reach and stretch higher and higher into the sky, as if you were touching the clouds. Reach all the way, and then pause. Then, slowly, smoothly, and gently return to an upright, seated position.

[Pause]

Sink more and more deeply into a pleasant state of relaxation.

[Pause]

Quietly open your lips, and let tension flow with every breath.

[Pause]

Let the flow of breath be as gentle as the flow of a quiet mountain stream.

[Pause 10 seconds]

[Breathing]

Take in a deep breath, filling your lungs completely.
Gently exhale.

[Pause]

Become more and more still.

[Pause]

Let the air flow out of your lips with every breath.

[Pause]

The only sound you hear is the quiet flow of breath and a quiet mountain stream.

[Pause]

Let your flow of breath be as gentle as a mountain stream.

[Pause 15 seconds]

[Imagery: Sitting on the banks of a mountain stream]

Now, quietly attend only to the image of sitting on the banks of a cool, refreshing mountain stream.

[Pause]

Become more and more still.

[Pause]

Your feet gently swing in the cool, refreshing water.

[Pause]

Tension flows down each leg, into your toes, and is dissolved and carried away by the water.

[Pause]

Quietly open your lips and let tension flow with every breath.

[Pause]

The flow of breath is as gentle as a mountain stream.

[Pause]

With every outgoing breath, let go of your worries over the past and future.

[Pause]

You can see the clear, sparkling water, smell its clean spray, and feel the warm sun on your skin.

[Pause]

Your mind becomes peacefully centered.

[Pause]

Time is like a river, each crisis passes and is forgotten.
Let yourself relax at your own pace; if your mind wanders from time to time, that's fine.

[Pause]

Attend with all of your senses to this beautiful, relaxing moment.

[Pause 1 minute]

[Meditation]

Quietly attend to the coming and going of the present moment.
If you are distracted, that's OK; simply return to your relaxation.

[Pause 5 minutes]

In this silent moment you realize that all things come and go. It is good. You are doing fine. It is time of deep inner peace and joy.

[Pause 1 minute]

Take in a deep breath.
And exhale.
Gently let go of what you are attending to.
With every outgoing breath, let your eyes slowly open to the outside world.
(This concludes the relaxation script.)

ADD ANTICIPATIONS OF SETBACK, REINFORCEMENTS, PAUSES AND SILENCES, AND TERMINATION SEGMENT

Evaluation of Your Script

Once you have written your script, it is useful to check for possible problems. Is it too long or too short? Are the instructions concrete and specific? Include every detail and leave very little to the imagination. Remember that you do not want to be concerned with filling in missing details or figuring out what ambiguous instructions mean. So instead of saying, "Do some yoga stretching with your arm," say, "Slowly, smoothly, and gently stretch and reach with the right arm." One instruction that is far too vague might be, "Imagine a cool pond and relax." This one is better: "Picture yourself next to a clear, cool pond. There is barely a ripple. The water is blue. The sky is clear without a cloud. You can feel a calm wind." Examine your script for any statements you question. Avoid statements like:

You will immediately recover from your cold.

You will find the answer to your problem.

You are now more relaxed than you have ever been before.

Frankly, you may not immediately recover from your cold, find an answer to your problem, or become more relaxed than ever. So avoid making promises you might not be able to keep.

Here are some examples of relaxation sequences that illustrate the script rules we have outlined. You may choose to use these as models when writing your own sequence.

Sample Relaxation Sequences

Example: Muscle Relaxation

Goal: General stress management
Unifying Idea: Detecting and releasing muscle tension

In this exercise, we are going to quietly look for and release sources of muscle tension. We will do this several ways, first by actively squeezing and letting go, then letting go as we exhale and release our breath, and finally by engaging in a special type of mental imagery. Note that we will shift from active to passive relaxation, not only in each exercise, but in the entire sequence.

Take in a deep breath, and make a tight fist.
Hold the tension.
Notice how tension feels.
And *let go*, gently letting out all the air. That's good.

[Pause]

Let the tension begin to flow out of your fingers.

[Pause]

Study the difference between sensations of tension and relaxation.

[Pause]

As your fingers become more relaxed, think the words, "fingers warm and heavy, fingers warm and heavy."

[Pause]

Attend to the sensations of relaxation as you sink into relaxation.

[Repeat Twice For Every Major Muscle Group]
This completes our muscle relaxation exercise.

And now we move to exercises that are more gentle.

Slowly take in a deep breath.

[Pause]

Notice any feelings of tension you may have.

[Pause]

And gently *let go.*

[Pause]

Let tightness flow out as you exhale.

[Pause]

Let the flow of air bring warmth and heaviness to your fingers, hands, arms, and feet as you sink deeper into relaxation.

[Pause]

Compare the subtle sensations of tension and relaxation.

[Pause]

It's OK to let yourself have feelings of warmth, tingling, or heaviness.
As we continue, our exercises become more and more passive and quiet.
Let your breathing continue easily and unforced.

[Pause]

Quietly attend to your hands and fingers.

[Pause]

Imagine a warm stream of air gently caressing your hands and fingers.

[Pause]

The flow of air dissolves your tensions and carries them away.

[Pause]

Very slowly and gently, the flow of air starts at your wrist and smoothes out remaining tension all the way to the fingertips. Picture tension as tiny wrinkles that are easily smoothed into relaxation.

[Pause 15 seconds]

See if you can tell the difference between very slight feelings of tension and relaxation.

[Pause 15 seconds]

Let yourself sink more and more deeply into a pleasant state of relaxation. Your mind focuses more and more on the calm you have created.

[Repeat for arms, back, shoulders, neck, face, legs, and feet]
Let yourself relax.
Quietly attend to the feelings you have created.

[Pause]

Gently open your eyes. Stretch your neck as you look around.
This completes our breathing relaxation.

Example: A Yoga Stretching Meditation

Goal: Recovery from a hectic day
Unifying Idea: A palm tree bowing in the wind

Imagine you are a palm tree standing by the ocean. As the wind blows, big waves crash against the shore. Each wave releases its tension as the water runs up and dissolves into the sand. The warm sun shines overhead, a source of life and energy for all the world.

[Pause]

A long, slow gust of wind sighs through the leaves.

[Pause]

Slowly, smoothly, and gently bow over and stretch completely.

[Pause]

Feel the stretch completely, all along your arms and torso.

[Complete stretch]

As the gust subsides, gently unstretch and release your tension.

[Pause]

You end your stretch and a wave crashes against the shore, releasing its energy into the sand.

[Pause]

The sun overhead bathes you in an ocean of peaceful clear light.

[Pause]

The wind begins to grow more gentle.

[Pause]

Even more easily than before, slowly reach up and stretch. Stretch all the way, barely rustling a leaf.

[Pause]

Gently return to your upright position, as a wave quietly releases its tension against the shore. At the end of the stretch, let yourself settle into stillness in the warm sun.

[Complete stretch. Repeat for neck, face, and legs]

Let yourself enjoy this relaxation. You have the capacity within for creating peace and calm. Let your mind attend to the good sensations you have created.

[Pause]

The waves have settled into quiet ripples lapping against the shore.

[Pause]

As you let yourself sink deeper into a pleasant state of inner calm, very slowly and easily rock back and forth to the easy rhythm of the waves.

[Pause 10 seconds]

Let your movements be so gentle that they barely stir the air.

[Pause 10 seconds]

You have few cares or concerns as you attend only to this rocking motion.

[Pause]

Quietly overhead, the sun continues to touch all with its delicate and gentle rays.

[Pause]

The wind becomes completely quiet and the ocean is still.

[Pause]

Let your body become motionless as you settle into a deeper calm.

[Pause]

It is good to let your mind center on the warm sun against your skin. It reminds you that you can trust your innermost thoughts and feelings.

[Pause]

Whenever your mind wanders, that's OK.

[Pause]

Gently return to the sun as it bathes you in peaceful life-giving light.

[Pause]

This is your meditation focus for the next five minutes.

[Pause 5 minutes]

Gently let go of what you are attending to. Attend to the sounds around you. What do you hear?

[Pause]

Slowly open your eyes, letting light in bit by bit. What do you see?

[Pause]

Take a deep breath and stretch.
This completes our yoga stretching meditation.

Example: A Creativity Exercise

Goal: Enhanced generation of ideas
Unifying Idea: The black stone

Take in a full, deep breath and quietly exhale.
It is time to put aside effort and deliberate thought. You are about to embark upon a journey into your mind.
Once again, take in a compete breath, and exhale, this time a bit more gently.

[Pause 10 seconds]

You will have an opportunity to ask a question that is important to you and then silently let answers come from an inner source of creativity.

[Pause]

Continue to breathe fully and easily. Let each breath become increasingly calm.

[Pause 10 seconds]

Take your time. There is no need to hurry. Let yourself become centered for your inner journey.

[Pause 1 minute]

Imagine you are at the edge of a forest. The air is calm with anticipation and the sun waits silently overhead. Occasionally the song of a bird echoes into silence.

[Pause 10 seconds]

In front of you is the opening of a cave. You slowly approach and gaze inside. A long flight of granite stairs descends into darkness.

[Pause]

Here is where your journey begins. Even though the cave is dark, you feel reassured. Calmly and confidently, you begin your descent. One step at a time.

[Pause]

A quiet voice starts counting down, from 5 to 1. With each number, you gently breathe in and out, and descend a step. With each number, you let yourself become more centered, more open to the possibilities ahead.

[Pause]

5

You breathe, and take one step.

[Pause]

4

[Pause]

It is safe to let yourself be completely free from the constraints of the outside world.

[Pause]

3

[Pause]

Your mind becomes increasingly clear.

[Pause]

2

[Pause]

The cares of the outside world seem so distant.

[Pause]

1

[Pause]

At the end of the stairs you encounter a mysterious dark shining stone, as clear as a mirror, reaching from floor to roof.

[Pause]

Let your attention become centered on the darkness ahead. It almost seems as though you were looking into the infinite expanse of space. The stone seems deep with mystery. It seems alive.

[Pause]

Quietly attend to the stone and gently ask your question. And simply wait.

[Pause]

Say nothing. Do nothing. Expect nothing.

[Pause]

A creative source deep within holds the potential for answering your questions.

[Pause]

Attend to what the stone has to reveal to you, in whatever way or form it desires.

[Pause 10 seconds]

Whenever the stone responds, you acknowledge by nodding silently.

[Pause]

Continue attending, without thinking or analyzing any response.

[Pause 10 seconds]

Whenever your mind wanders, that's OK. Gently return.

[Pause]

This is your focus for the next 10 minutes.

[Pause 10 minutes]

Gently let go of what you are attending to.

[Pause]

Slowly acknowledge the stone and turn away.

[Pause]

You slowly begin climbing the stairs, step by step.

1

You climb closer to the surface.

2

You can hear the noises of the world outside.

3

Feeling quiet and peaceful, you approach the opening.

4

All around you is bright with sunlight.

5

Gently open your eyes.

Take a deep breath.

This completes our creativity exercise.

Brief Sample Relaxation Sequences

Here are some shorter examples adapted from another book of mine (Smith, 1992).

Example: The Pond

I imagine myself floating in a warm, soothing pond. I see wonderful things all around—green trees; the pure blue sky; and delicate, silky clouds. I can smell the clean, calm water, and hear it lapping gently against the shore and my body. It is a magical pond, one that supports me perfectly.

I very gently squeeze and shrug my neck and shoulders. Body heat and tension flow out and dissolve into the water. My body feels light, relieved of the cares and concerns of the day.

The water supports me like a feather. I attend to the easy flow of breath, in and out. Tension floats away with each outgoing breath. Gentle ripples float away on the water.

As I settle into stillness, I attend to the peaceful dome of sky above, the broad expanse of blue, pure and intense. There is nothing to do but watch the clouds lazily float by. All seems right in the world. My cares and concerns seem so distant and unimportant in the peaceful clear blue light of day.

Example: Healing Powers

I open myself to healing powers within. I imagine these powers as a warm energy, like a glowing fluid. I squeeze and let go in order to release blocks to the healing flow of this energy. As I stretch, I open pathways for this energy to flow to parts of my body most in need . . . my heart and my immune system. I feel my heart beating more and more slowly, and the warm blood carrying healing energy throughout my body. As this energy dissolves tension and disease, I imagine myself gently breathing out poisons and breathing in healthful, healing air.

Example: The Flight of the Bird

I am a bird perched on the sill of a window. Night is approaching and the sky is growing cool and dark. I stretch my arms out like wings, and raise them higher and higher. With a gentle gust of air, I imagine myself floating into the air, supported by the wind as I lower my arms. I float higher and higher, far away from my concerns. And with a deep, refreshing breath, I float far above the clouds. All around is the dark blue dome of night sky. I feel completely safe and sheltered, yet open to the vast mystery of the universe.

Example: The Candle

My tensions are like the hard wax of a candle. I squeeze my neck, and the flame ignites. I let go, and the tension begins to melt like wax, flowing away. Every time I squeeze and let go, more wax melts. My mind becomes centered on the single flame of the candle. I gently open my lips and breathe out very gently, barely causing a ripple. With each outgoing breath, even the slightest tensions dissolve and float away. I calmly attend to the candle. It reminds me that the spirit of life within me keeps on burning in spite of my tensions.

Example: The Teacher

I feel close to my spiritual teacher, a very old man from centuries ago. I slowly stretch my arms open, and feel he is lovingly embracing and supporting me. As I unstretch and relax, I feel him holding and caring for me. Throughout life I am supported by powers unseen.

Example: The Garden

I imagine I am a flower in an immense and beautiful garden. I gently bow over and stretch; dew drops of tension flow off and dissolve into the soil. Relieved from the weight of tension, I slowly reach up to the sky and open the warm light of the sun. I can see the vast garden of flowers around me. I breathe in slowly and deeply; I smell the fragrances of life. I feel I am one with all life around.

Example: The Field of Wheat

I am sitting in a field of wheat. An ocean of golden grain flows with the wind. I reach high into the sky and stretch with every ounce of my being. I greet and celebrate the bounty around. I take in a deep breath and can smell the rich harvest around. Then I bow over, stretching my back. I touch the grain below and can smell the earth. I feel one with the world. I then simply stand and let myself become more and more centered. I calmly attend to a single grain of wheat. The warm sun sinks into my skin. I feel nurtured by the life and bounty around.[2]

EXERCISE 14.1 *Applying Script Principles*

If you are in a coping team, see if you can figure out which script-writing ideas are used in Sue's script as well as the examples presented at the end of this chapter. Can you find examples of:

Relaxation goal

Unifying idea

Deepening words

Deepening affirmations

Coherence

Anticipation of setbacks

Relaxation reinforcements

EXERCISE 14.2 *Writing Your Own Script*

Coping team members should each write their own scripts, then share them with other members.

Compare relaxation goals and exercise selections, as well as similarities and differences between scripts. Members can offer suggestions to each other for modifying scripts.

EXERCISE 14.3 *Advanced Deepening Strategies for Your Script*

If you enjoyed the process of writing a relaxation script, you might want to consider the following instructions for deepening your script even further.

[2]Adapted from J.C. Smith, *Spiritual Living for a Skeptical Age: A Psychologial Approach to Meditative Practice.* Copyright 1992, New York: Insight Press, an imprint of Plenum Publishing Company. pp. 35, 46–48.

One way is to introduce *deepening imagery*, that is, imagery that changes in a direction of increased focus, letting be, and openness (see Chapter 12). Note how the following imagery is initially complex and active, and then becomes more focused, and reflects greater letting be and openness.

> You are on a quiet beach. As you sit up and look around, you notice the blue water and sky. The sun is directly overhead, its warm rays dissolving tension in your body. You can feel a breeze and hear the soothing waves splash against the shore. As you become more relaxed, you recline on the beach. Your attention narrows to the sky above, and the peaceful clouds floating by. There is nothing you have to think about or do. Simply attend to the clouds and nothing else. All sorts of thoughts and images may come to mind, and that's OK. Simply let them come and go, and return your attention to the graceful clouds.

The use of *metaphors* can enhance relaxation by symbolizing both concrete exercises procedures and relaxation philosophies. A swaying tree can signify a yoga stretch or the philosophical statement "Flow with the here and now." Crashing ocean waves can signify the exhalation of breath, or a commitment to "let go of that which cannot be changed." Such metaphors are, in a sense, more abstract than exercises, and more concrete than philosophies. Since they exist at an intermediate level of abstraction, they can be used to foster transitions from concrete exercises to affirmations of philosophies. This is illustrated here:

Stretch and unstretch your arms.

Stretch and unstretch your legs.

With each stretch you are like a tree swaying in the wind.

Stretch, unstretch, and sway in the wind.

A tree sways in the wind, firmly rooted in the earth, yet flowing with the moment.

Remember how you, firmly supported by the ground of life, can flow with the moment.

If more than one exercise is selected, *deepening transitions* can be introduced between each. Such transitions reinforce the thought that your exercises are not an arbitrary assortment, but lead deeper and deeper into relaxation. A transition phrase can be as simple as this:

We have now completed one exercise and will move on to an exercise that is even more passive and calm.

Another way to deepen relaxation is to introduce a *relaxation countdown*. Start with any number, usually 5 or 10, and slowly count back to 0. Each count is associated with deeper levels of relaxation. Begin to count backwards from 5 to 0. With each count, let yourself become more and more relaxed.

Tense up.

And let go.

We begin with 5.

Attend to the sensations of relaxation.

4

Let the tension slowly begin to flow out of your muscles.

3

Notice the difference between tension and relaxation.

2

Let your muscles become more and more fully relaxed.

1

Let go of any feelings of tension you may feel.

0

Enjoy the feelings of relaxation you have created.

Countdowns can be woven into just about any approach to relaxation. For example, in stretching and breathing sequences, they can be incorporated with unstretching and exhalation. Imagery provides the richest opportunity for countdown relaxation. Here the actual content of an image can change or reflect increasing depth. This is illustrated by the following image of floating into the clouds:

You begin by resting on earth and become so relaxed that you begin to float.

5

As you let go of your tensions, you become lighter and lighter.

4

Your mind centers on the peaceful sensations of floating and relaxation.

3

You float higher and higher. The houses and trees below become smaller and smaller. Your everyday pressures and concerns seem so distant.

2

As you approach the peaceful soft clouds, your mind feels more and more free, more open to the possibilities of relaxation.

1

You float into the clouds, completely without effort or concern. You settle into a deep and comfortable state of relaxation.

Interpersonal Stress

It is not difficult to see that stress is most commonly caused by personal interactions. Whether it be poor communication between lovers, excessive demands from a supervisor, inadequate feedback from a teacher, or just one of the many insults and confrontations encountered in the course of living, people create stress. In this and following chapters we focus on interpersonal topics of shyness and loneliness, requests and conflict, anger, negotiation, and reaching out to others.

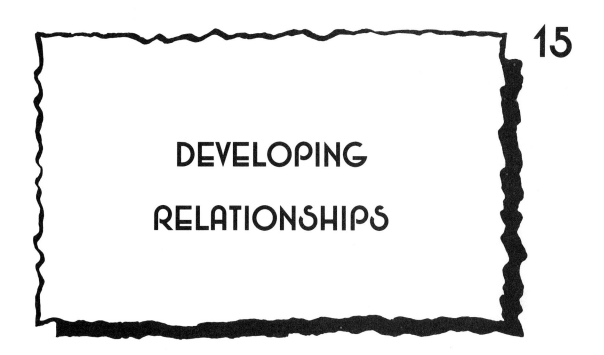

15 DEVELOPING RELATIONSHIPS

Target Coping Skills

- Initiating, maintaining, and ending a conversation; exploring possible relationships

Purpose

- Elimination of loneliness and shyness
- Initiation of friendships
- Development of friendships you already have
- Ability to cope with rejection, loneliness, and shyness

Example

Louis lives a lonely life. He has started college miles away from home and knows no one. He is afraid to meet others because they might reject him, or not become his friend. To deal with this general problem, Louis focused on a specific subgoal—meeting others. First he listed all the places he could meet people, including church, class, and the school cafeteria. Then he assigned himself the task of learning to "break the ice" by going to one of these places at least once a day, introducing himself to at least one person, and then treating himself to a good dinner. Once comfortable with this, he expanded his task to pursuing a conversation with at least one person a week. Here, he practiced asking questions, listening, commenting, and sharing his thoughts and feelings. This task also gave him good practice in learning to deal with his big fear, rejection. He learned to practice his people-meeting skills and to treat rejection as opportunities to grow.

CUE → COPE → REWARD summary: TRIPS TO "MEETING PLACE" → INTRODUCTION TO AT LEAST ONE PERSON → DINNER

Many people find the process of meeting others and getting to know them very stressful. Avoiding the stress of forming and nurturing relationships can lead to feelings of loneliness, depression, and helplessness. One can feel lost, out of control, and overwhelmed. But our fundamental belief is that such feelings are often a cue that a pragmatic, problem-solving perspective may be in order.

It can be useful to differentiate *social loneliness* and *emotional loneliness* (Russell, Cutrona, Rose, & Yurko, 1984). Social loneliness is the result of not feeling part of a group. As a result, you do not have anyone to share your feelings or common experiences. Emotional loneliness is caused by "breaking up" with friends and lovers, and the rejection or loss of others.

The first step in dealing with both types of loneliness is to look at your interpersonal goals and to determine how you try to meet them. Are your goals and attempts to cope working? Are they simple, concrete, and realistic, or vague, overemotional, and abstract? Here are some examples:

I want people to like me.

I want to have a lover.

I want to have a friend in whom I can confide.

I want all of this right away. I can't stand being alone.

I should be more attractive. I can't do anything about it because I am unattractive.

I should be more outgoing. I don't have an outgoing personality.

Others just don't want to get to know me.

I just don't know.

Can you see why these goals and coping attempts are not working? The goals ask for too much too soon. Relationships grow over time; one does not instantly acquire friends and lovers. And the coping attempts are vague. It is more sensible to look for specific *situations* that could contribute to the development of relationships. Look at your goals and coping attempts in these four situations:

- Initiating a conversation
- Maintaining a conversation
- Ending a conversation
- Dealing with rejection

Initiating a Conversation

Shy and lonely people lack the skills to start conversations. Often they are preoccupied with making a good impression and are fearful of rejection. This can lead to an avoidance of meeting people. But avoidance is hardly a good way to combat loneliness and shyness.

Where are the people I want to meet? Whom do you want to meet? Where can you go to meet them? How do you approach them? It can be dangerous to become preoccupied with such questions, especially the question of whom you want to meet. Many people develop an idealized image of someone they would like to know, their "knight in shining armor" or "princess in flowing gowns." The problem is that few people meet such idealized expectations, and often it is difficult to judge the type of person best suited to you. A more sensible strategy is to meet people first and then decide which relationships you would like to continue.

We now have our first simple and concrete stress situation—finding good places to meet others. This is a goal that makes sense. Can you brainstorm possible answers?

How do I break the ice? Imagine you are at a party. You see someone by the punch bowl you would like to meet. But you are not sure of what to say. As a result, you never meet the person. Different versions of this same situation are probably repeated numerous times every day. You sit on the bus next to someone you would like to know. At work or school, you would like to meet the person at the desk next to yours. You are playing basketball and want to meet a certain person in the locker room. What do you say? How do you act?

One of the easiest ways to break the ice is with an *opening line*, a question or comment you have thought of beforehand. Researchers have actually studied the types of opening lines that work and do not work (Kleinke, Meeter, & Staneski, 1986). Here are some of the better ones:

"Hi."

"Can you give me directions to ______?"

"Can you help me with ______?"

"Did you see (name a movie or TV show)?"

"Have you read (name an article or book)?"

"I feel a little embarrassed about this, but I'd like to meet you."

"That's a very pretty sweater (shirt) you have on."

"You have really nice hair (eyes)."

"Since we're both sitting alone, would you care to join me?"

"Is it OK if I sit with you?"

And here are some openers that do not work:

"I'm easy. Are you?"

"I've got an offer you can't refuse."

"What's your sign?"

"Didn't we meet in a previous life?"

"Your place or mine?"

"Is that really your hair?"

"You remind me of a woman (man) I used to date."

"Isn't it cold? Let's make some body heat."

Can you see why the good lines are more likely to work? Some are innocuous and nonthreatening. They give the other person a very easy way out. Others are simple, direct, and honest statements. What about the openers that are less likely to work? Generally, they come across as insincere and flippant. Avoid such abrasive opening lines.

In addition to opening lines, questions are a good place to begin. Make your questions open-ended; it doesn't make sense to ask a question that can be answered by a single yes or no. You can see how the following opening lines go nowhere:

You: "Hi. Do you live here?"
Other person: "No."
You: "Hi. Hot enough for you?"
Other person: "Yes."
You: "Hi. Do you like this bar?"
Other person: "No."

Open-ended questions are invitations for the other person to say something about themselves. For example:

"That's an interesting design on your shirt. Could you explain what it means?"

"What do you think of this place? I'm sort of new here."

"What kinds of things do people do here to have fun?"

And avoid some of the mistakes shy people often make in attempting to break the ice. These include:

Deliberately filling the air with talk, not giving the other person time to respond

Making self-conscious put-downs in an attempt to appear more likable

Standing next to someone, grunting a perfunctory ice-breaker, "Oh, hi," and waiting for the other person to take over.

And before breaking the ice, think of some back-up or follow-up lines. What will you say when the other person responds? What will you say if they do not respond? What will you say if they respond only a little? Opening lines can be much more than formal ice-breakers. They are ways you, and the other person, can quickly scan common interests and any interest in continuing the conversation.

Research also suggests that men meeting women should be aware that women prefer a quiet and nonthreatening approach. The "macho approach" so popular in the movies does not usually work in real life. If you have difficulty taking rejection, innocuous lines are safer. For women who want to meet men, first it is important to know that it is OK to be the first to break the ice. There is no need to wait around. There is less research on men meeting men, and women meeting women; here, be direct, or at least innocuous.

When breaking the ice, your body language can turn people off or invite them to get to know you better. Look the other person in the eye. Lean towards them. Smile. Speak loud enough so that they can hear you.

Maintaining a Conversation

You are sitting with a stranger and have just introduced yourself. The other person says nothing. Should you continue? What is the other person thinking? What next? It is not enough to initiate a conversation. Like lighting a log in the fireplace, you need to nurture the budding flames. In general, others have suggested (Conger & Farrell, 1981; Greenwald, 1977; Kupke, Calhoun, & Hobbs, 1979):

Look for signs the other person wants to continue. The best sign is when they give you "free information" about themselves, their thoughts and opinions. Free information goes beyond a simple, perfunctory yes and no. Also, some obvious body signals can tell you if the other person wants to continue. Are they smiling? Facing you? Looking in your direction (or away, at someone else)?

Pay attention to what the other person is saying. Restate their key points to show you understand and are "with them." Show that you accept and understand the other person's feelings. It can help to empathically restate the feeling (see Chapter 18).

When you pursue your conversation, do not be afraid to talk. Shy people often believe that once they break the ice, the other person can take over. In fact, conversations are most successful and enjoyed when both people talk about the same amount of time.

Conversations grow as people share more and more information about each other. As you tell the other person about how you feel, what you like, what you think, and what you do, you invite them to respond in kind. But avoid premature intimacy (sharing with a stranger about your recent divorce, operation, emotional turmoil). It can be useful to think through ahead of time some safe topics you are willing to discuss. These might include: your home town; your thoughts on marriage and children; your plans at school; your career plans; what you like to do in your spare time; an interesting thing you have just done this week; and your hobbies.

You, or the other person, may well grow tired of a particular topic while the other may want to continue. It is your right to suggest changing the topic. Often honesty is the best policy:

"Would you mind if we talked about something else?"

"You know, I just thought of something I would like to share with you."

At the very least, provide some polite signal or transition that indicates that you are changing themes. If the change is abrupt, a small apology can be useful.

"I know I'm changing the topic, but something just came to mind I would like to discuss with you."

Ending a Conversation

When you are ready to quit talking, or sense the other person is ready, then it is time to politely stop the conversation. There are several ways of doing this:

Summarize what you have talked about ("We seem to agree on who should be president.")

Simply state your readiness to leave. ("Well, we've had quite a talk. It is now time for me to go.")

Show your interest in the other person. ("I've enjoyed this conversation and would like to meet with you again.")

Politely excuse yourself. ("I've enjoyed talking with you. I must excuse myself to go home and . . .")

State your plans for what to do next. ("I've planned to do some shopping today. I need to go.")

Dealing with Rejection One of the reasons shy and lonely people avoid making conversation is fear of rejection. But your goals for meeting others can determine how you view rejection. If you see each person you meet as an opportunity to explore someone else and practice coping skills, then rejection becomes part of exploration and growth. However, if your goal is to fall in love with the other person, make the other person fall in love with you, or form a connection to advance your career, then you may be setting yourself up for a distressful rejection. Once again, as we emphasized at the beginning of this chapter, start with sensible goals for meeting others.

EXERCISE 15.1 *Meeting Places*

In this exercise, you and your coping team should first think of as many settings as you can where it might be possible to meet others. Be creative, not critical. The first goal is to produce quantity, not quality. Then select which seem to be the most sensible places. You can extend this exercise over a week and, as a homework assignment, ask your friends for ideas, or ask people like bartenders, ministers, coaches, teachers, and waitresses. Go to places that reflect your interests, such as movie theaters or museums.

EXERCISE 15.2 *Getting Practice in Meeting Others*

Often a good way to develop your skill at using "openers" is to try them in safe situations with strangers you are not anxious about meeting. Try talking to strangers on the bus, at school, or at work. Report to your coping team on the success of your experiments. Try role-playing meeting others in your coping team. The team members can imagine they are having a party, sitting at a bar or waiting for a bus. You can practice initiating and maintaining conversation in preselected situations.

EXERCISE 15.3 *Pursuing a Conversation*

Practice maintaining a conversation with a person in your team. Pick a "safe" person that in actual life you are not trying to meet. See if you can maintain a conversation for 10 minutes. Then extend it to 15 minutes.

EXERCISE 15.4 *Barriers to Developing Relationships*

Use exercises 7.1 and 7.2 to consider thoughts and attitudes that might get in the way of meeting and getting to know others. Think of a situation in which you wanted to meet, or get to know someone better, but did not. What thoughts were going through your mind? How did they interfere? How were they irrational or maladaptive? What replacement thoughts can you think of?

16

MAKING REQUESTS, SAYING NO, AND DEALING WITH CONFLICT

Target Coping Skills

Effectively stating a request, including the facts and your feelings that make your request one that should be taken seriously; outlining the benefits if your request is met, and the costs if it is not

Purpose

- Requests for raises
- Refusal of reasonable sounding requests you just do not want to honor (such as helping friends or relatives and volunteering for community organizations)
- Attempts to get someone else to change their behavior, if it is hurting or offending you
- Requests in any difficult interpersonal situation

Example

Patricia wants to ask her boss for a raise. She has worked well for over three years without a single raise and feels her contributions to the company are being slighted. The moment she sees her boss, she approaches him and offers a reasonable proposal: "I have worked for this company for over three years and have not received a single raise. This frustrates me since I see others getting raises. I guess my sense of fairness tells me that good performance should be rewarded, and I feel I am performing well. I would like to put in a request for a raise this year. Frankly, getting a raise will make me feel much better about working here and 'going the extra mile' to do a good job." After making the proposal, she praises herself for making such a good presentation.

CUE → COPE → REWARD summary: CONVERSATION WITH BOSS → PROPOSAL FOR RAISE → SELF-PRAISE

The DESC Script

Sharon and Gordon Bower (1976) have developed a very useful system for managing many stressful situations. They call it the "DESC script," which stands for "DESCRIBE-EXPRESS-SPECIFY-CONSEQUENCES." Here's how it goes:

Describe the other person's behavior that is a concern for you.

Express what you feel and think about this behavior.

Specify explicitly what changes you would like in this behavior.

Spell out the *Consequences* to both of you if your concern is, or is not, resolved.

In working on a DESC script, use D'Zurilla's (1986) rules for defining a problem (Chapter 3). Present your facts in concrete, specific terms. Focus on what is factual, not opinion or emotion. Use the "W" questions:

Who is involved?

What happens (or does not happen) that bothers you? What needs and wants are being frustrated? What goals are in conflict?

Where does it happen?

When does it happen?

Why, as far as you can tell, does it happen?

What is your response (actions, thoughts, and feelings)?

Can you see how this DESC script does not meet these rules?

Situation: Matt and David work together in a local paint shop. Over the last few weeks, Matt has taken few days off to visit his sister. David has had to take over Matt's work in order to ensure that customers would not leave dissatisfied. During lunch one day, Matt turns to his partner and unexpectedly makes a request: "Dave, would you mind taking over for the rest of the day? I have to go." David has had enough. He feels taken advantage of and feels Matt is not doing his share of the work. Here's what he says:

> Matt, you just aren't carrying your weight around here. I've just about had it. I would really appreciate it if you would be a bit more responsible.

If you look at what Matt said carefully, it is possible to identify Describe, Specify, and Consequence lines. However, they do not follow good problem-defining rules. The problem, as well as David's emotional response and request, is vague and imprecise. Here is the same exchange rewritten in a more effective way:

> Matt, last Tuesday, Thursday, and Friday you did not show up for work. I had to complete your painting contracts for you. And now you are asking me to do this again. This is beginning to irritate me. I feel it is unfair that you ask favors for nothing in return. Please, the next time you can't do your work, give me at least a week's notice, and make arrangements to do some of my work in exchange. If we can work this out, I'll feel more comfortable working with you, and helping you out.

Notice how this response is specific and concrete. It gets to the point, and is not distracted by needless emotionality or pointless personal attacks. It focuses specifically on the problem behavior, and makes a specific request.

The DESC script was introduced as a way of dealing with conflict. Portions of it can be used in a variety of interpersonal stress situations, as can be seen in the following examples:

Meeting and Getting to Know Someone

(Situation: For several weeks you have been sitting next to a newcomer at work whom you would like to meet. You have not said anything yet and are very frustrated.)
Describe: I notice we've been sitting next to each other for about a month and haven't met.
Express: I'm feeling a little frustrated; I like to know the people I work with.
Specify: My name's Jack. What's yours? I would like to get to know you better.
Consequences: I notice you are new here. If I can help you out in any way, please let me know.

Expressing Positive Feelings

(Situation: You have had a roommate for about six months and really enjoy his company. However, you have not told him this, fearing his reaction.)
Describe: I've been keeping something to myself I would like you to know.
Express: I like having you as a roommate. You're fun to have around.

Expressing Opinions

(Situation: You are having lunch with your supervisor from work. She makes a point about which you disagree. You hesitate expressing your opinion.)
Describe: I hear you saying that productivity might increase if we work on Saturdays.
Express: I'm not really sure this is a good idea.

Assertive Rights

One problem people have with DESC scripts is the feeling that they do not have the right to use them. People often feel they are being too "pushy," "insensitive," or "demanding." If such thinking is a problem for you, it can be useful to stand back and consider your *assertive rights.* An assertive right is a course of action you reasonably and realistically have the right to pursue. Jakubowski and Lange (1978) have identified eleven such rights:

1. The right to act in ways that promote your dignity and self-respect as long as others' rights are not violated in the process
2. The right to be treated with respect
3. The right to say no and not feel guilty
4. The right to experience and express your feelings
5. The right to take time to slow down and think
6. The right to change your mind
7. The right to ask for what you want
8. The right to do less than you are humanly capable of doing
9. The right to ask for information
10. The right to make mistakes
11. The right to feel good about yourself. (pp. 80–81)

These rights might seem perfectly obvious. However, when people hesitate to express their thoughts, feelings, and wants, it is often because they feel they do not have the right to be assertive. They may think:

"I can't say no when a friend asks to borrow my car. She would think I'm selfish."

"I can't let my wife know how depressed I am. She just wouldn't understand."

"They want me to tell them right away what I think of their plan. I can't tell them I want time to think. They'll think I'm indecisive."

"I can't change my mind after I told them what I think."

"I can't let myself make a mistake on this project. I would feel just terrible."

Each assertive right is actually a response to an irrational belief or expectation. To believe that you should never promote self-respect, say no, express your feelings, take time to think, and change your mind is simply unreasonable. One of the first steps in learning to be more assertive is to identify and challenge such irrational denials of "perfect rights," and to affirm what rights you can reasonably claim. It is thinking:

'I can't say no . . . now, wait a minute. I have my needs and rights. I don't *have* to go along with what others want, just as they don't *have* to go along with what I want."

"I can't let my wife know how depressed I am . . . now, wait a minute. I'm only human. Everyone has feelings, both good and bad. After all, she's my wife. She should know how I feel."

"I can't change my mind . . . but, no one's perfect. I have good reasons for changing my opinion, and I want to be honest."

"Everyone is out to get me. No one cares for me . . . I'm going to have to fight for myself, and attack others to get ahead."

In a more general sense, a person's denial of his or her assertive rights is a *rationalization* for being too passive. A rationalization is an excuse, an attempt to convince ourselves to avoid dealing with a problem assertively. Here are a few common rationalizations:

"I'm afraid I'll displease others" (Rational response: "I can please everyone all the time.")

"I can't be assertive; maybe the other person will retaliate" (Rational response: "Let's think this out. Just how likely is it that the other person would really retaliate?")

"I can't express my negative feelings. I would feel so guilty if I hurt the other person's feelings." (Rational response: "Is there a way of saying what I feel without hurting the other person? Perhaps this is a situation where some feelings of hurt just can't be avoided.")

"Everyone is out to get me. No one really cares what I think. It's a waste being reasonable. I have to fight and attack." (Rational response: "It's unreasonable to believe that everyone is so hostile. Some people are, and some aren't. It might be more useful for me to first find out where the other person stands rather than presume their hostility.")

In sum, learning to deal with stress assertively involves changing both thoughts and behaviors. It involves knowing what to say, what to do, and what thoughts and beliefs are rational and useful.

Nonverbal Assertiveness

We have focused on the thoughts and actions associated with assertive coping. However, often what we do not say is as important as what we do say. If you stand with shoulders slumped and eyes downturned while making a request, your body language conveys a nonassertive message no matter what you say. Similarly, if you shake your fist and grit your teeth while making what you think is a reasonable request, you body is conveying an aggressive message. These points are covered in greater detail in Chapter 17.

EXERCISE 16.1 *Composing a DESC Script*

In the space below, write a DESC script for a stressful situation. If you are in a coping team, have team members evaluate how concrete, specific, and realistic your script lines are.

SITUATION:

DESCRIBE:

EXPRESS:

SPECIFY:

CONSEQUENCES:

EXERCISE 16.2 *Assertive Rights*

Think of a situation in which you were not assertive. Can you think of any assertive rights you were denying yourself? Thinking realistically, what assertive rights do you have in such a situation? This exercise can be done as a group project.

EXERCISE 16.3 *Barriers to Making Requests, Saying No, and Dealing with Conflict*

Use Exercises 7.1, 7.2, and 7.3 to identify and analyze thoughts that might interfere with your willingness to make requests, say no, and deal with conflict. Think of a situation in which you failed to make a reasonable request, say no, or deal with a conflict.

What thoughts were going through your mind that interfered?

How were they distorted, unrealistic, or maladaptive?

What were the costs and payoffs of these thoughts?

What are some realistic and practical replacement thoughts?

17

DEALING WITH YOUR ANGER

Target Coping Skills

- Differentiating aggressive, assertive, and passive behavior
- Learning to express anger appropriately and effectively
- Learning to restrain potentially self-destructive anger
- Finding alternatives to anger

Purpose

- Response to verbal attacks
- Control of impulsive anger in oneself
- Anticipation of potentially dangerous "anger" situations
- Plan for remedies when you do get out of control
- Instruction on recovery from anger

Example

James tends to "blow up" at work at the slightest provocation. Later he regrets his behavior, when it is usually too late. Using the ideas of this chapter, he learned to identify early warning signs of his anger—shaking hands and heavy breathing. Recognizing these signs gave him enough time to plan and use alternative responses that would "defuse" his anger and help solve underlying problems. Part of this involved repeating to himself the phrase, "Let's be careful. How can we solve this reasonably?" He added to his skills by learning how to "cool off" during an angry episode, and to manage anger from others. After successfully practicing, he indulged in bragging to his friends about his success. CUE → COPE → REWARD summary: SHAKING HANDS AND

HEAVY BREATHING → "LET'S BE CAREFUL" REMINDER → BOAST TO FRIENDS ABOUT SUCCESS

When considering anger, it is useful to begin by making some distinctions. First, aggression is destructive *behavior*, whereas anger is an internal *feeling*. While it is often appropriate to monitor and control aggressive behavior, feelings cannot always be controlled. It is important to realize that the feeling of anger can serve as a useful warning sign that you may be about to engage in aggressive or self-destructive behavior.

Aggressiveness, Assertiveness, and Passivity

People often confuse aggression with assertiveness, and equate an absence of aggression with passivity. The difference emerges when we consider the goals of these behaviors. Assertive goals are to effectively, honestly, and directly state what is on your mind. It is appropriately expressing your thoughts, feelings, wants, and beliefs. Aggressive people may also want to express themselves. However, they often do so at the expense of others. To the simple goal of honest expression, they add the goals of dominating, hurting, humiliating, and manipulating others.

The difference becomes even more clear when we contrast aggressive and assertive roles. The aggressive role is one of a controller, manipulator, owner, and even parent. The assertive role is one of an adult, peer, equal, and colleague. Thus, when some people say they are being "aggressive" they actually mean "assertive," if they are expressing their feelings in an appropriate and adult manner.

Aggressive people sometimes fear that lack of aggression means the same as passivity. Here too, there are important differences. Passive people simply do not state what is on their minds. Their goals are to keep thoughts, feelings, wants, and opinions to themselves, to give in to others, please others, avoid trouble, and "be a nice person." They take on the role of a helpless person, a child or a victim.

Aggressive, assertive, and passive behavior each have their own body language, as can be seen below:

Aggressive Behavior

Eye contact: Staring; looking down; looking away impatiently

Facial expression: Clenching teeth; pursing lips; sneering smile

Voice and speech: Talking too loud or rapidly; being sarcastic; remaining silent

Posture: Standing too close or far away; leaning over or standing too close to the other person

Gestures: Making a fist; pointing a finger; shaking head; placing hands on hips

Assertive Behavior

Eye contact: Making direct eye contact; looking away when appropriate

Facial expression: Reflecting honest feelings, interest or concern; looking serious but not threatening

Voice and speech: Speaking in firm, warm, clear and expressive voices; placing proper emphasis on key words so they are clearly understood

Gestures: Emphasizing key words without intimidating or dominating

Passive Behavior

Eye contact: Looking up, away, or down; blinking frequently; staring ahead with glazed eyes

Facial expression: Constant smiling to hide true feelings and "not make waves"; smiling or laughing when expressing negative feelings; swallowing or clearing throat

Posture: Slumping over; turning away; standing stiff or too far away

Gestures: Fidgeting; covering mouth with hand; nodding head inappropriately; pacing or shifting; restless fidgeting (playing with tie or hair)

Examples of Aggressive, Assertive, and Passive Behavior

It is not difficult to think of straightforward examples of aggressive, assertive, and passive behavior. Most fall into the following categories (Smith, 1991):

Direct Communication and Interaction

Meeting and Getting to Know Someone

Aggressive: "You look cool. My place or yours tonight?"
Assertive: "I noticed you were standing alone and thought I would introduce myself."
Passive: Standing against the wall, hoping someone else will introduce him or herself.

Expressing Positive Feelings

Aggressive: "You're lucky I like you. I usually can't stand freshmen."
Assertive: "You know, I like you."
Passive: "Oh, I don't mind it too much when you're around."

Expressing Sadness, Fear, or Anxiety

Aggressive: "Sure, I've got a big job interview coming up. Someone like you just can't realize how talented I am."
Assertive: "I've done my best preparing for this job interview. It still makes me anxious, but I think I will do OK."
Passive: "This job interview? I just can't do things like this."

Expressing Opinions

Aggressive: "I voted for Jones, and you're stupid to vote otherwise."
Assertive: "I decided to vote for Jones."
Passive: "I just don't know how to make up my mind. Tell me how you'll vote."

Requests, Refusals, and Negotiation

Making requests

Aggressive: "Give me your book."
Assertive: "I left my book at home. Could I borrow yours for a time?"
Passive: "Gosh, I left my book at home. I see you have a book. I wonder how I'll study."

Saying no

Aggressive: "No, I won't give to your church. Stop bugging me."
Assertive: "No, I have decided not to give to your church this year. Thanks for asking, and good luck in your fund-raising campaign."
Passive: "Maybe I'll give. Just leave your literature here so I can mail my money in sometime later."

Negotiating

Aggressive: "Listen, this is how we'll do it. You give me the $10 and I'll let you borrow my car."
Assertive: "We can solve this problem if we get our heads together. To begin, I am willing to let you borrow my car, but I need something in return."
Passive: "Well, OK, I guess you can have my car."

Conflict Situations

Standing Up for Yourself in Impersonal Situations

Aggressive: (Someone slips in front of you in the grocery checkout line.) You say, "You're a real pig, aren't you?"
Assertive: "Excuse me, I was standing there."
Passive: "Oh, hi. I didn't know you were standing here."

Offering Negative Feedback

Aggressive: "You're just out of line. Can't you get anything right at work?"
Assertive: "Last week you left work without putting your tools away. Tonight, I see you haven't put them away again. I must ask you to put your tools away."
Passive: "Getting a little messy around here, isn't it?"

Expressing Anger

Aggressive: "You stupid fool!"
Assertive: "You broke my bicycle without telling me. That makes me angry."
Passive: "I'm a little concerned about our relationship is going."

Dealing with Negative Feedback

Aggressive: "You can't tell me to study harder for the exam. Do you think you own me?"
Assertive: "I know I failed the last exam. But it doesn't help when you just tell me to study harder."
Passive: "I'll try to do better."

Dealing with Hostile Criticism and Anger

Aggressive: "You call me stupid? Well, you're a meathead!"
Assertive: "I don't believe this name-calling is getting us anywhere."
Passive: "Excuse me, I have to go to the bathroom."

Sometimes it is difficult to differentiate assertive, aggressive, and passive behavior. The following examples highlight some finer points:

Example: Mable has let Joan borrow her accounting text. Joan has not returned it for a month, even though Mable has asked for it three times. To let Joan know her feelings, Mable borrows her hair dryer, and does not return it. Mable figures, "This way, Joan will get the idea."

Analysis: This is a special form of passive behavior called passive-aggressiveness. Here, Mable does not directly express her wish—to have her book returned. Instead, she "gets back" in a passive way.

Example: Felix has just broken up with his girlfriend and feels hurt and vulnerable. Right now, he could use a little support and reassurance. His good friend Fred decides that assertive honesty is the best policy and blurts out, "Gosh, Felix, you've got only yourself to blame. Your shirts are at least four days old, you need a haircut, and you typically wait for your date to call and ask you out."

Analysis: The point here is not whether or not Fred is right. There is a time and place to be assertive, and a time and place to keep quiet. Given Felix's vulnerability, perhaps Fred should have kept his feelings to himself for a while. This is an example of inappropriate assertiveness.

Example: Sherrie is an older college student who appears to be the victim of what seems like nonstop harassment. Every noon she eats lunch in the school cafeteria. Mildred, a younger student, sits with her and begins talking and asking inappropriately personal questions. At first, Sherrie was passive. She politely nodded her head, but continued eating without responding. Week after week Mildred continued. Sherrie then decided to be assertive, turned to Mildred and calmly explained, "I do not want to hurt your feelings. But for the last three weeks you have been sitting with me and asking me questions about my boyfriends, choice of deodorant and medical problems. This embarrasses me, especially since I want to eat lunch alone. Mildred, I'm going to have to ask you to find someone else to eat with. That way, I can eat in peace and you can find someone you really enjoy talking to." Mildred did not hear this clear request and continued sitting with her. One day she sat next to Sherrie and started asking her about her personal life. Mildred replied with a simple request: "Please leave me alone. I want to be by myself. I've had it with you."

Analysis: Sherrie eventually resorted to aggressive behavior. However, it is clear that she chose this behavior and was aware of its consequences. This example illustrates that aggression, like assertiveness and passivity, can have its place.

There is a time and place for aggression and for anger. Indeed, one can assertively express anger. However, the effective coper has a choice and can decide when to be aggressive, assertive, or passive. Some feel they do not have a choice. The key to learning to deal with aggression is learning when to use it, when not to use it, and how to deal with it in others.

1→2→3 COPE and Anger

The 1→2→3 COPE system works particularly well in learning to gain control over your own aggressiveness. Identify situations in which you are likely to be inappropriately aggressive. Then look for the cues that come before and the costs and benefits that come after. Aggression management involves modifying cues and consequences, and finding effective replacements for aggression.

Consequences

When people engage in aggressive behavior, they often consider only the short-term gain, the fact that they "got it off their chests," or exerted control. However, any behavior has costs as well as benefits. What are the costs of aggressive behavior? Often they obscure their points with emotion and additional demands. They reduce the possibility that the other person will respond assertively, that is, as a mature equal seeking to resolve an honest difference. Think of a recent stress situation in which you responded aggressively. What were its costs and payoffs?

Triggers of Aggression: Critical Moments and Warning Signals

What are the "triggers" likely to set off unproductive aggression on your part? Look for immediate critical moments and early warning signs. These include physiological signs within yourself, such as muscle tension, a knot in the stomach, a clenched fist, grinding teeth, and a pounding heart. Are you assuming an aggressive posture, standing too close to the person, "staring them down," arms crossed in a tough position? In addition, look for behavior you see in others that may be provocative. Also be aware of aggressive thoughts you may be entertaining ("Boy, I'll teach them a lesson." or "That is it. I can't take any more.")

Coping Thoughts and Actions

A central part of most aggression-control programs (Novaco, 1975) is planning ahead. Once you have made a decision that you want an alternative to responding aggressively, and have identified useful critical moments and early warning signs, what can you do? Some simple anger reducers can be applied after critical moments. These include:

- Breathing deeply
- Counting backwards from 20 to 1
- Engaging in a pleasant scene that you have thought of beforehand
- Practicing any self-relaxation exercise (Chapters 10–13)

If you have a bit more time, it can be useful to think ahead of some useful thoughts and behaviors. Novaco suggests the following for different stages of a provocation:[1]

Preparing for Provocation

This is going to upset me, but I know how to deal with it.

What is it that I have to do?

I can work out a plan to handle this.

I can manage the situation. I know how to regulate my anger.

If I find myself getting upset, I'll know what to do.

There won't be any need for an argument.

Try not to take this too seriously.

This could be a testy situation, but I believe in myself.

Time for a few deep breaths of relaxation. Feel comfortable, relaxed, and at ease.

Easy does it. Remember to keep your sense of humor.

[1]Adapted by permission from Novaco, R. W. (1975). *Anger control: The development and evaluation of an experimental treatment.* pp. 95–96. Lexington, MA; D.C. Heath.

Handling Impact and Confrontation

Stay calm. Just continue to relax.

As long as I keep my cool, I'm in control.

Just roll with the punches; don't get bent out of shape.

Think of what you want to get out of this.

I don't need to prove myself.

There is no point in getting mad.

Don't make more out of this than you have to.

I'm not going to let him get to me.

Look for the positives. Don't assume the worst or jump to conclusions.

It's really a shame that she has to act like this.

For someone to be that irritable, he must be awfully unhappy.

If I start to get mad, I'll just be banging my head against the wall, so I might as well just relax.

There is no need to doubt myself. What he says doesn't matter.

I'm on top of this situation and it's under control.

Coping with Arousal

My muscles are starting to feel tight. Time to relax and slow things down.

Getting upset won't help.

It's just not worth it to get so angry.

I'll let him make a fool of himself.

I have a right to be annoyed, but let's keep the lid on.

Time to take a deep breath.

Let's take the issue point by point.

My anger is a signal of what I need to do. Time to instruct myself.

I'm not going to get pushed around, but I'm not going haywire either.

Try to reason it out. Treat each other with respect.

Let's try a cooperative approach. Maybe we are both right.

Negative leads to more negatives. Work constructively.

He'd probably like me to get really angry. Well, I'm going to disappoint him.

I can't expect people to act the way I want them to.

Take it easy; don't get pushy.

Reflecting on the Provocation

(When conflict is unresolved)

Forget about the aggravation. Thinking about it only makes me upset.

These are difficult situations, and they take time to straighten out.

Try to shake it off. Don't let it interfere with your job.

I'll get better at this as I get more practice.

Remember relaxation. It's a lot better than anger.

Can I laugh about it? It's probably not so serious.

Don't take it personally.

Take a deep breath.

(When conflict is resolved or coping is successful)

I handled that one pretty well. It worked!

That wasn't as hard as I thought.

It could have been a lot worse.

I could have gotten more upset that it was worth.

I actually got through that without getting angry.

My pride can sure get me into trouble, but when I don't take things too seriously, I'm better off.

I guess I've been getting upset for too long when it wasn't even necessary.

I'm doing better at this all the time.

These steps are not engraved in stone. In working with people who have problems with aggression, I find that it is useful to think through the unique steps each individual seems to go through

. In thinking through the steps your aggression takes, it can be helpful to fantasize in your mind an aggressive encounter. Or, you might role-play an encounter with your coping team.

EXERCISE 17.1 *Phases of Aggression*

What phases of aggression do you experience? What are some useful coping strategies for each?

EXERCISE 17.2 *Analyzing Aggressive, Assertive, and Passive Behavior*

Think of examples of assertive, aggressive, and passive behavior. If you are in a coping group, see if you can identify how these behaviors differ with respect to their goals, consequences, and nonverbal behavior.

EXERCISE 17.3 *Identifying Steps in an Anger Situation*

In your coping team, select a situation in which you expressed anger inappropriately. First analyze your goals and role. Then, break the situation down into steps. Examine your coping options for each step.

EXERCISE 17.4 *Angry Body Language*

In your coping team, select an anger situation that one member has experienced. This person, or others, can role-play the situation. Team members identify the nonverbal behaviors indicating anger. To extend this exercise, team members can consider appropriate alternative thoughts and actions. These can then be role-played.

EXERCISE 17.5 *Cost/Benefit Analysis*

In deciding the appropriateness of an assertive course of action, it is often useful to weigh the short- and long-term consequences of your actions. In this exercise, select a situation in which you have difficulty responding assertively.

First, what were the specifics of this encounter?

What happened?

Who was involved?

What did the other person(s) do and say?

What did you do and say?

What stress symptoms and emotions did you feel?

Now, describe an appropriate assertive response to this situation.

In the spaces that follow, list the costs and benefits of your response. Follow each short-term cost or benefit with the words "short-term." The remaining costs and benefits we will assume to be long-term.

Your Assertive Option:

Costs

Benefits

18

DEALING WITH AGGRESSION

Target Coping Skills

- Identifying hidden aggression; managing verbal aggression

Purpose

- Response to others with hostile or manipulative behavior
- Success in making your point, or solving a problem, when others appear to be working against you
- Success in getting back on track after someone has diverted your attention through their aggression.

Example

Jonah works in a secretarial pool and frequently feels under attack. Specifically, she has a problem with Delilia, one of her co-workers. Often, Delilia will display such subtly aggressive behavior as ignoring Jonah's complaints, changing the topic, and offering superficial apologies. On one occasion, Delilia initiated a rather heated and emotional argument about who is responsible for answering the phone. Using the ideas in this chapter, Jonah replied by noting Delilia's anger: "I can see this is really upsetting you." She pointed out the impact the anger was having by responding, "However, your outburst isn't solving anything. It's just upsetting people in the office." Jonah concluded with a suggestion that got to the point: "Let me suggest we put our feelings aside and try to solve this in a mature way." Later, Jonah sorted out how this was an improvement over going along with Delilia's attack. CUE → COPE → REWARD summary: DELILIA'S INITIATION OF ARGUMENT → JONAH'S

RECOGNITION OF DELILIA'S ANGER → JONAH'S APPRECIATION OF IMPROVED WAY OF COPING

Dealing with unprovoked aggression from others can be a problem for many people. Aggression is rarely pleasant, and can contribute hurt feelings and confusion. From a problem-solving perspective, aggression can distract you from your goals, or provoke you to deviate from sensible coping solutions you have attempted.

Most forms of aggression are fairly obvious. People who physically attack you, yell at you, call you names, or verbally abuse you are obviously aggressive. But people are often subjected to aggression without realizing it. It can be useful to examine the more subtle forms aggression can take, as well as the different ways aggression can have an impact on you (Bower and Bower, 1976; McMullin, 1986).

Aggressive Behaviors

Distraction The other person may prevent you from making your point or solving a problem by distracting your attention with incidental or irrelevant comments. Examples:

"Oh, what kind of after-shave is that you are wearing?"

"You're so sexy when you're mad."

"Gee, you're getting pushy."

- Possible payoff to other person: They prevent you from talking about what you want to discuss. They confuse or upset you.
- Possible cost to you: You do not get to finish what you were planning to say or do. You feel hurt, put down, or ignored.

Blanket Denial Here, the other person simply refuses to accept what you are saying without further discussion. Examples:

"I never said I would take you home from the party."

"All of your concerns just aren't true."

"It just isn't an issue. We don't have to talk about it."

- Possible payoff to other person: They shut off discussion of a potentially uncomfortable topic; denier takes on the role of controller or manipulator.
- Possible cost to you: You feel you have exaggerated a point or made a mountain out of a molehill. You do not make your point.

Discounting Similar to denial, this form of aggression involves minimizing the importance of your point. Examples:

"Come on, lighten up!"

"I was just trying to do my best. Why are you so upset?"

"What's the big upset all about?"

- Possible payoff to other person: They seem calm and in control.
- Possible cost to you: You wonder if you are taking things too seriously and are less inclined to push your point.

Victimization How is it aggressive when another person avoids an issue that is important to you by playing hurt, or taking on the role of a helpless victim? At the least they are taking control of the discussion and manipulating it without your consent. Here are some examples:

"You brought up a point that really makes me feel bad. Why do you hurt me so?

"I've been sick recently and just haven't been doing my best."

"Everything is going wrong for me. And then you bring up this."

- Possible payoff to other person: They maintain manipulative control of a discussion; they gain sympathy from you.
- Possible cost to you: You may compromise or "give in" out of guilt feelings.

"Yes . . . Yes . . . Yes" One quick way to interrupt your coping efforts is for the other person to profusely, and apologetically, agree with whatever criticism you may offer. Examples:

"How could I be so stupid? Of course, you're completely right. We don't have to talk about this any more."

"OK, you're right and I'm wrong. That's that. End of discussion."

"Oh, I'm so, so sorry. I can't apologize too much for what I've done. I really feel so badly about what has happened. Really, I am extremely sorry."

- Possible payoff to other person: They shut off discussion of an uncomfortable issue; they win sympathy from you.
- Possible cost to you: You may feel you have been too hard on the other person and compromise your original criticism.

The Silent Treatment Here, you make a point to another person and they simply ignore you. Variations can include refusing to answer phone calls or making a point and then walking away.

- Possible payoff to other person: By doing very little, they get to avoid a problem.
- Possible cost to you: Because you are unsure of how the other person is responding, you become confused and do not persist; the other person may make you feel your point is just not worth considering.

Making a Joke of It Here the other person tries to "laugh off" a problem by turning it into a joke or cute comment. Examples:

"Well, you didn't like my criticism of your make-up. Better watch it—your face is getting so red you'll melt your eye shadow."

"Why did I forget to call? Well, I just wanted to see if you were dating anyone else."

"Hey, I can push you when I want. It helps build muscle."

- Possible payoff to the other person: They get to show that they are "above it all."
- Possible cost to you: You feel your point is unimportant; you feel guilty returning to a serious issue after a good laugh.

"Psychologizing" Here the other person makes unfounded inferences concerning your hidden feelings, motives, and plans. This can include bringing up "psychological history" such as your childhood, early character or relationship with your parents. Examples:

"Just like a woman (or man) for you to say that."

"Why are you getting so paranoid?"

"You have problems getting close to others; that's why you don't want to see me."

- Possible payoff to other person: They establish themselves as an "astute observer" who knows more than you do about your own behavior.
- Possible cost to you: You doubt your own motives; you become preoccupied defending yourself.

Arguing Others can avoid problems by arguing about some irrelevant or secondary point. Examples:

"You're claiming that it is my turn to clean the apartment. I don't recall that cleaning included sweeping the floors."

"I don't take good care of the things I borrow from you? What do you mean by 'borrow,' anyway?"

"I know I promised I would study with you over the weekends. But talking on the phone is a form of study, isn't it?"

- Possible payoff to other person: They define the topic under discussion.
- Possible cost to you: You become preoccupied in an endless "no win" discussion.

Blaming Here, another person tries to divert your attention by blaming problems on you, or on someone or something else. Examples:

"You can't expect me to always return your calls when you call so often."

"It's hard for me not to yell at the children when you're causing me so much stress."

"Sure, I'll get more work done—when you quit interrupting me."

- Possible payoff to other person: They offer an excuse for their behavior.
- Possible cost to you: You question if your original goals are legitimate.

Managing Aggression from Others

People behave aggressively in many ways. Not only do they physically and verbally attack, but they manipulate, play guilt games, ignore what you are saying and jokingly use sarcasm. Remember, whenever someone is not treating you as a peer or equal, or when they seem to want to dominate, manipulate, hurt, or attack, they are behaving aggressively. Jakubowski and Lange (1978) list three goals that make sense when you are confronted with aggression:

- Get to the source of the problem.
- Try accomplish your goals.
- Limit the other person's aggressive behavior.

Getting to the Source of the Problem

Simply responding empathically can help defuse a potentially aggressive situation and help get to the source of a problem. This involves temporarily ignoring the hostile content of someone's remark, and observing the upset, pain, and hurt that you see (Chapter 18). For example:

Barry: You left early last week and I ended up having to do extra work. I really resent it when you do this.
You: I can understand how angry you must have felt.
Betty: My birthday was last week and you didn't do a thing. You must take me for granted. I really feel like I've been put down.
You: Yes, I can see you're upset that I didn't remember your birthday.

There are several payoffs with empathic listening. First, you communicate your genuine interest in going halfway in seeking a resolution. You set the tone for a more calm and reasonable dialogue. And you show that you care about the other person.

Another strategy is to ask for a clarification. Often angry people confuse the issue with emotion, or add issues to the original complaint. In getting to the complaint, you might acknowledge or ignore the emotional content and focus on what the problem might be. ("Yes, you are really angry about this, but please help me out. Just what did I do that created such a problem?") Here, it can be very helpful to use a concrete, specific, and realistic problem-solving approach suggested in this book. Ask for a sample situation—a concrete illustration of a specific problem behavior. Which goal was not being met?

Finally, let the other person know the message you are hearing. This can help the other person fine-tune their criticism and present it in a way more conducive to practical problem-solving. For example, you might say:

You: Now, what you've just told me is that I am stupid, careless, and can't get anything right. The impact on me is that I simply don't know what to do to make things better.
Other person: Well, I didn't mean to put you down so much. But to be honest, your laziness really gets to me.
You: I'm lazy. That's an awfully big accusation. I don't know where to begin to understand what you mean. Should I work harder at school? On the job? With the kids? I'm confused.
Other person: No, no. I'll get to the point. Last night you didn't clean up our shared office as you promised. As a result, I felt upset and let down.

In letting the other person know the impact of their statements and behavior, it can be useful to look for what Bower and Bower would call the DESC script hidden in their message (Chapter 15). A DESC script is a simple and effective way of making a complaint. It consists of four steps:

Describe the objective behaviors that make up a problem.

Express your feelings and thoughts about these behaviors.

Specify your wishes for concrete and realistic change.

Outline the *consequences* (that is, the costs and payoffs) if the request is or is not met.

If you can get another person to rephrase their aggressive attacks into a DESC script, you help defuse a potentially serious problem and get to its source.

Accomplishing Your Goal

What is it that you want out of this encounter? In what way is the other person's aggression interfering with this goal? Here are a number of techniques Jakubowski and Jakubowski suggest for accomplishing your objective:

- Ignore the other person's aggressive comments and simply persist with what you want to say.
- Simply and directly point out the irrelevance of what the other person is saying and return to your main point.
- Put the aggression aside as an issue that can be dealt with later; return to your goal.

Limiting the Effects of Aggression

Sometimes it is best to attempt to limit aggressive behavior. This can be the case when it is clear that an aggressive encounter is going nowhere, or that it is escalating. Here are some suggestions:

- Ask questions to prompt the other person's awareness of their aggressive behavior.
- Behave in a calm, problem-solving manner, in direct contrast to the aggressive behavior being displayed.
- Provide direct and specific negative feedback.
- Treat a put-down as a neutral comment (ignore the emotional component and focus on what might be true).
- Sort out fact from judgment and interpretation. Focus on the facts.
- Announce your intent to escalate your assertions, and wish for a contract to end the aggression.

EXERCISE 18.1 *Identifying Hidden Aggression*

If you are in a coping team, each member should think of an example of subtly aggressive behavior. Other team members can identify how it is aggressive, as well as the payoffs of such behavior to the other person and the costs to you.

EXERCISE 18.2 *Managing Aggression*

Think of an example in which you handled aggression well. Which strategy did you use? Can you think of any additional strategies?

EXERCISE 18.3 *Role-Playing Aggression*

First, the coping team should select an aggressive situation to role-play. The coping team then forms two groups—one the aggressors and the other the victims. The aggressor team selects one person to engage in verbal aggression, while the victim team selects someone to be the recipient. In separate rooms (or in different corners of the room), each team works on the strategies their selected role-players will use. What forms of aggression (nonphysical, please) will the aggressor use? How will the defending team respond? After this preparation, the aggressor and victim then role-play the selected situation. After role-playing, both teams can comment on what happened, suggest improvements, and role-play again.

19

LEARNING TO NEGOTIATE

Target Coping Skills

- Negotiating a resolution to a conflict.

Purpose

- Situations in which both parties to a conflict are willing to compromise and approach negotiation in a fair, problem-solving frame of mind
- Generation of conditions conducive to effective negotiation
- Identification of impediments to negotiation
- Tactics for deadlocked discussions

Example

Matt and Marti are working together on an important class project. However, they have serious differences on how to proceed and they decide to negotiate. First, they select a quiet and neutral setting, a picnic table in the park. They agree beforehand to think through their most important priorities. The discussion starts with Matt and Marti both stating their own positions and checking if they understand each other clearly. They then proceed with a give-and-take negotiation, with each making compromises, until a final resolution is reached. They reward themselves by going out for a drink. CUE → COPE → REWARD summary: STATEMENT OF OPENING POSITIONS → NEGOTIATION → TRIP OUT FOR A DRINK

A friend once presented a puzzle: "What happens when two people have equally legitimate but different goals? What prevents a psychological tug-of-war where both dig their feet deeper and deeper in the sand?" Obviously such complex problems often call for a complex strategy for dealing with stress—negotiation.

Negotiation is a part of life. It is rare that we have the same wishes and opinions as our friends, families, and co-workers. Indeed, what a dreary world it would be if we did think alike! The healthy and adult way to deal with differences is to talk about them honestly and sincerely. Put differently, negotiation is the process of two or more people dealing assertively with each other.

Blocks to Negotiation

Often irrational and self-defeating beliefs interfere with effective negotiation. Perhaps the most important is the tendency to approach conflict with a *win-lose* strategy. That is, the goal to achieve one's own goals and defeat the other person as in combat or competitive sports. In negotiation, the goals are a little different. Here, you adopt either a *win-win* or *compromise* strategy. You recognize the possibility that, with honest, adult communication, both parties may well achieve their goals, or both may have to give a little in order to get what they want.

A wide range of other beliefs can interfere with resolving conflict:

Conflict is bad and should always be avoided.

There is only one right answer (usually yours).

All conflicts must be solved.

Compromise means that you are weak.

Compromise always means that someone will get hurt.

The winner gets all in a negotiation.

The first step in effective negotiation is to be clear as to your own expectations concerning negotiation. Conflict is not necessarily bad and can lead to desirable growth and change. It is indeed an expression of strength to be willing to honestly negotiate. And a willingness to negotiate means a willingness to compromise.

Preparing for Negotiation

Psychologist Arnold Goldstein has written much on how to negotiate (Goldstein & Keller, 1987; Goldstein et al, 1976; Goldstein & Rosenbaum, 1982). The first thing to keep in mind is that effective negotiations do not just happen. They require some preparatory conditions to "set the stage." Here are four that Goldstein recommends:

1. *Remain calm.* High levels of stress can interfere with your ability to think and solve problems effectively. If you are extremely angry or upset, select a time to negotiate when you are feeling relatively calm. You might even practice relaxation before negotiating.
2. *Think out your priorities and desires beforehand.* Begin negotiation with some sense of what you want and what is important. You may have to compromise, so recognize where you can be flexible. Select goals that are fair and simple. Do not overwhelm the other person with goals that are excessive.
3. *Pick a private and neutral setting.* Negotiation is more likely to work in a setting where there is little chance of interruption. When others are present, both parties may want to "play to the audience" and avoid compromise or attempt to save face. Also, pick a place that is neutral for both of you. A person negotiating on home turf (their home or office, for example) is more likely to be assertive and less likely to compromise.

4. *Negotiate face-to-face.* It is important to see the other person when negotiating. Because both of you can see each other's facial expressions and gestures, the chances of misunderstanding are reduced.

The Five Steps of Negotiation

Goldstein and Rosenbaum (1982) suggest five negotiating steps to facilitate the actual process of negotiation, as follows:

1. *State your position.* Begin with a moderate opening position in which you demand neither too much nor too little. How you state your position can do much to establish helpful levels of trust, toughness, and cooperativeness.
2. *State your understanding of the other person's position.* Negotiations often fail because one person simply fails to understand what the other person really wants. This is a risk especially when levels of tension are high. A simple way of avoiding this problem is to state your understanding of the other person's position. You may even try to put yourself in the other person's shoes and try to see the world as he or she sees it. Such efforts often have additional payoffs. You help establish a cooperative rather than combative atmosphere and you invite the other person to understand your position.
3. *Ask if you have stated the other person's position accurately.* "Checking things out" is an important part of constructive communication. It is often not enough to simply assume you understand each other. Be open to the real possibility of misunderstanding. Communication can also be helped by repeating points that are particularly difficult and putting your ideas in the other person's language. Most important, make it clear that it is important to you that you understand and be understood.
4. *Listen to what the other person has to say.* This might seem like an obvious part of negotiation, but it is often overlooked. When tensions are high, negotiating parties are often tempted to make a firm and final "position statement" and wait to see if it is accepted or rejected. But there can be no negotiation if there is no give and take. And for this to happen, you need to be a good listener. Do not interrupt or tune out what you do not want to hear; do not speak impulsively without thinking, or bring up distracting, irrelevant points. Goldstein suggests that you attempt to listen as though you have to summarize to someone the other person's point.
5. *Propose a compromise.* When both of you have made your positions clear and you understand each other, it is time to explore a compromise. Remember that, in a compromise, each person gives a little in order to get something. The best compromise is the win-win solution in which both parties figure out how both can come out ahead.

Compromising is a process of demanding and conceding, giving and taking. Earlier, you set your goals and priorities. Now you know what the other person wants. With this information in mind, suggest compromises that are direct, specific and concrete, and well reasoned.

Obviously the shrewd negotiator does not "give away the store." Recognize that both of you have priorities, easy concessions you can make early on, and more costly concessions you save for later. A shrewd negotiator also does not "burn bridges," that is, offer concessions as final promises rather than tentative and provisional suggestions. If the other person does not follow through with acceptable concessions, you may well have to withdraw yours.

Breaking Deadlocks

We started this chapter with a question—what happens when simple assertiveness does not work? The same question can be asked concerning negotiation. What can be done when both parties have reached a deadlock?

First, make sure you have not created problems by setting up needless barriers. For example, one obstacle to negotiation is the *self-fulfilling prophecy*. Here, your expectations of what the other person might say and do actually cause the other person to behave that way. Here is one example:

> Michael has made an appointment to see his History teacher about a low grade he received on the final. The night before he spends considerable time worrying about this appointment. He thinks, "This teacher must be out to get me. She never smiles at me in class. I bet she thinks I'm lazy. Boy, I'm going to have a hard time." The next day, Michael meets with his teacher. Thinking she must be irritated, he trembles and blurts out a challenge, "I know you think you're too good for us, but I want to ask about my grade." Somewhat startled by this attack, the teacher stands back, frowns, and says, "Michael, I'm not sure what your problem is." Michael takes this as more evidence that his teacher does not like him and becomes even more tense.

In this example, Michael's preconceived and distorted notions concerning his teacher caused him to act in a defensive and belligerent way. Understandably, she reacted with a certain degree of irritation, confirming Michael's expectations. Even though she may not have been angry at first, Michael established a self-fulfilling prophecy.

Often roadblocks are set up by needless provocations. If things are not going smoothly in a negotiation, ask yourself if you are needlessly attacking the other person, leaving them little room to maneuver. Are you avoiding the main issue, distracting the other person, or trying to save face? Remember, negotiation is not combat. Two equals with legitimate concerns engage as adults in the process of give and take.

If it becomes clear that a deadlock has been reached, Goldstein suggests increasing bargaining room. See if you can change your terms or demands or increase your flexibility. Both parties may have to take additional risks, and you can test if this works by proposing an additional compromise. In addition, sometimes the other person may avoid accepting your compromise simply to save face. Make it clear that you are both making compromises, and that making a compromise is not a sign of defeat or weakness. You might remind the other person about the terms on which you both agree. Finally, sometimes deadlocks require that you stop negotiating. You might take a temporary break or even seek a third person to mediate your conflict.

Contracting

Just as there are many factors that can interfere with your completion of an individual stress management exercise, much can get in the way of fulfilling a negotiated solution. For example, you or the other party may have second thoughts. Perhaps the original agreement does not work as expected, or creates unexpected costs. Contracts can be useful for following through with a negotiated solution.

We have noted that a good contract should have the following features:

1. *What will you do?* Spell out in concrete, and specific terms what you plan to accomplish. Make your goals limited, simple, and realistic. It is better to attempt one thing rather than everything.
2. *When will you do it?* Specify target dates for when you will begin and complete your task.

3. *How will you reward yourself?* Pick a reward that fits the task, one that is not too generous or stingy.
4. *When will you reward yourself?* Be sure to give yourself a reward immediately after you achieve your goal. State when in your contract.
5. *How will you penalize yourself for not completing your task?* Select an appropriate and specific penalty for not completing your specific goal.
6. *What bonuses might you award yourself?* Bonuses are special rewards for when you achieve more than you contracted for (or complete your goal before the time stated in your contract). State what your bonus will be, and when you will award it to yourself.
7. *How will you keep a record?*

Signature: ______________________________ Date: ______________

With only a few modifications, this contract can be applied to negotiated solutions (Goldstein & Keller, 1987). First, to minimize misunderstanding, the contract should be in writing. It should be fair. Ambiguities, hidden meanings, and "fine print" should be avoided. Contracts should be public, to serve as a reminder for each party to meet the terms. Finally, contracts should be reviewed periodically so that reasonable adjustments can be negotiated and added.

The Assertive Reply

Negotiations do not always succeed. There are times when the differences between parties are too great to be resolved. You may well have to agree to disagree. You may have to settle for the goal of expressing how you feel and simply live without a solution. A useful way of concluding such a conflict is to apply the Bower and Bower DESC script (1976). There are four components to this approach:

Describe the problem.

Express what you think and feel about it.

Specify what concrete behavioral changes you desire.

Outline the *consequences* if these changes occur.

When applied to unresolvable conflict, a useful DESC script might state:

Describe: We have negotiated this problem for three days. Both of us have made a reasonable attempt to offer solutions and compromises. But we still haven't reached a solution.

Express: I feel very frustrated when I can't negotiate a solution. But I also feel resigned that perhaps that is how it will have to be.

Specify: Let me suggest that we stop our negotiations and accept that we both have legitimate, but irreconcilable, differences.

Consequences: I would like to leave feeling that at least we made our best effort to resolve our differences and that we still respect each other.

A variety of other strategies are often mentioned in books on coping. Most consider what happens when the other party refuses to engage in negotiation and insists on being aggressive. If this happens, consider the suggestions in Chapter 18.

EXERCISE 19.1 *Evaluating Negotiation Strategies*

Think of a situation in which you attempted to negotiate a compromise with a friend. First, describe the specifics. Who was involved? What happened? When or where did it happen? What were your goals? What were the goals of the other person?

Now, which of the following describe your negotiation?

Preparing for Negotiation

1. Did you remain calm?
2. Did you think out your priorities and desires beforehand?
3. Did you pick a private and neutral setting?
4. Did you negotiate face-to-face?

The Five Steps of Negotiation

1. Did you state your position?
2. Did you state your understanding of the other person's position?
3. Did you ask if you have stated the other person's position accurately?
4. Did you listen to what the other person had to say?
5. Did you propose a compromise?

Thinking back over what happened, how might you have improved your negotiation strategy?

EXERCISE 19.2 *Beliefs That Get in the Way*

In this chapter we listed a few of the dysfunctional beliefs that can get in the way of effective negotiation. These include:

Conflict is bad and should always be avoided.

There is only one right answer (usually yours).

All conflicts must be solved.

Compromise means that you are weak.

Compromise always means that someone will get hurt.

The winner gets all in a negotiation.

Can you think of any others that apply to you or to people with whom you have negotiated?

EXERCISE 19.3 *Role-Playing a Negotiation*

This exercise involves practicing your negotiations skills with your coping team. It involves these steps:

1. Select an issue you feel is appropriate for negotiation. Consult with your coping team. Is it an appropriate topic of negotiation or a no-win problem? Is the topic realistic, concrete, and specific or vague and emotional?
2. Select some other person(s) to play the role of the other party.
3. Let the person(s) who are playing the other party know what they will be thinking and saying. What are their goals? What are their tactics?
4. Now the other party leaves the room and privately works on a negotiation strategy. They should try to anticipate what points you might bring up and how they should respond. They should clearly identify their goals and how they might compromise.
5. While the other party is planning their strategy, you do the same with the help of your coping team.
6. You and the other party meet with your coping team and select an appropriate (imaginary) setting for your negotiation. Use the suggestions in this chapter.
7. You and the other party begin negotiation while your coping team observes. Continue negotiation until a solution is reached or a deadlock is encountered.
8. You, the other party, and your coping team discuss the negotiation in terms of the principles in this chapter. Which principles were followed successfully? Which were not? How might the negotiation have been improved? How might it have been more realistic? How might you have handled possible setbacks and deadlocks?

20

DEVELOPING EMPATHY

Target Coping Skills

- Listening with empathy

Purpose

- Clear understanding of what another person is thinking and feeling
- Clear and effective communication to another person of what you hear them saying
- Enhanced communication and minimized misunderstandings

Example

Claire and Charles are living together. One night Charles comes home and is clearly upset. However, he is having trouble talking about his problem. Throwing his books on the table, he blurts out, "That stupid team. Why did I even think of trying out for basketball?" Claire responds empathically, "Charles, you're really upset. Something went wrong with the team you were going to try out for today." Inside, she breathes a sigh of relief that she broke the ice and is getting to the root of the problem. Charles, feeling that Claire is clearly interested and understands, begins to talk about how he was rejected for the team he had worked so hard to join. Eventually, he talks about his feelings of frustration and anger. After about an hour, feeling a lot better, he thanks Claire, "Thanks for being here with me and letting me unload. It was really helpful." CUE → COPE → REWARD summary: ANGER TOWARDS "THAT STUPID TEAM" → EMPATHY FROM CLAIRE → RELIEF OF TENSION

In this chapter we're going to do something a little different. Instead of looking at another way of directly managing or preventing stress, we will look at the support we can offer others through empathy and the support we can obtain from others. You might wonder what do these topics have to do with stress management? A great deal.

Empathy

Empathy is understanding and communicating your understanding of the thoughts, feelings, and wants of others. It is getting into the other person's shoes. Such empathy is essential for effective assertiveness, negotiation, and conflict resolution. If another person knows you want to understand, he or she is more likely respond in a mature manner. By using empathy, you can forestall possible misunderstanding. In a slightly different light, your empathic understanding of others can help them deal with stress better. Similarly, when looking for help, it is a good idea to find someone who knows how to listen empathically.

In trying to be helpful, people all too often miss the mark and end up doing more harm than good. Take a look at the following example. Dorothy is a college student and is having problems with her mother. Here is her complaint:

Dorothy: My mother just doesn't listen to me. I want to spend the weekend with a friend, and mother objects. She wants me back by 10:00 every evening. This really gets to me. I'm 21 and can make my own decisions. Sometimes I just feel like screaming.

Nonempathic Responses:

Mothers are mothers!

Well, you feel like screaming!

Oh.

Gee, I really understand.

Well, it sure looks like you have something of a conflict with your mother. It's not unusual for young adults to want to "leave the nest" while parents still want them home as children. Such conflicts are normal and are a part of growing up. Sometimes a good talk is what is needed.

How old is your mother? Do you live with her?

You should respect your mother. After all, she is getting on in years. You'll get over it.

You'll understand how your mother feels when you grow up and have children.

None of these responses is particularly empathic. Although quite possibly sincere, they are in fact:

Clichés

Parroted repetitions of the obvious

Vague, incomplete reactions

Attempts at make-believe understanding

Lectures

Interrogations

Judgments

Advice

Condescending or patronizing responses

Empathy is none of these. It is, once again, accurate understanding and communicating what another person thinks, feels, and wants. Here is our example, once again, with empathic responses.

Dorothy: My mother just doesn't listen to me. I want to spend the weekend with a friend, and mother objects. She wants me back by 10:00 every evening. This really gets to me. I'm 21 and can make my own decisions. Sometimes I just feel like screaming.

Empathic responses:

I sense you really feel frustrated over being treated like a child.

It irritates you when your mother doesn't let you do what you want.

You are a mature adult, and it upsets you when your mother doesn't recognize this.

Barriers to Empathy

In learning to be empathic, try to identify some of the barriers that can get in the way of listening. You can, for example, become preoccupied with yourself and your own needs so that you do not hear what the other person is saying. Gerry Egan (1982) has identified the following common barriers:

Attraction. If you are preoccupied with how attractive or unattractive the other person is, you are less likely to hear what the person is saying.

Your physical and emotional state. It is important to recognize when you are fatigued, emotionally upset, or under stress. You are less likely to be empathic.

Overeagerness. Trying too hard can get in the way. It is easy to become so involved with trying to figure out good empathic responses that you actually become less empathic.

Identification with the other person's problem. If the other person is dealing with a problem that is bothersome to you, this may distract you from accurately hearing what the other person is saying.

Prejudice. Our society clearly condemns prejudice because of race, nationality, sex, and religion. However, many of us harbor silent prejudices and stereotyped attitudes based on social status, political beliefs, sexual attitudes and lifestyles. Prejudices prompt us to make premature conclusions concerning others and we fail to understand how they really think and feel.

Primary-Level Accurate Empathy

Egan (1982) has identified two levels of empathy: primary-level and advanced accurate empathy. Primarily-level accurate empathy means "communicating *initial basic* underlying of what the client is feeling and of the experiences and behaviors underlying these feelings" (p. 87). The goal is not to probe deeply for profound psychological interpretations. Just say what you hear. What feelings are being expressed? What facts, opinions, or perceptions form the content of the other person's point? Here are some examples:

Other person: I came home from work late at night and was tired and frustrated. Nothing went right. Every suggestion I made was ignored. And to top it off, I let out my feelings to my roommate, who just continued watching TV. He didn't even grunt. This really burned me up.

Empathic understanding of feeling: You feel irritated that people just weren't listening.

Empathic understanding of content: Both the people at work and your roommate ignored what you wanted to say.

Other person: We've been seeing each other for nearly two months. I'm feeling a bit confused. I'm not sure where our relationship is going, and I'm afraid we might be getting too close too fast. I would like to spend this weekend by myself. I need the time.

Empathic understanding of feeling: You seem confused and uncomfortable about how close we might be getting.

Empathic understanding of content: You need a break this weekend. You need the time for yourself.

Note again that primary-level accurate empathy can focus on feelings ("You're irritated, confused") or factual content ("You've been ignored, want to be alone.").

Advanced Accurate Empathy

In trying to understand other people, we often have to get below the surface and clarify hidden meanings. Advanced accurate empathy focuses on both what the person is actually stating, and what you think they are implying or partially expressing. It is not "playing psychoanalyst" and unearthing deep and profound explanations ("You say that because you have deep conflicts with your parents"; "You have questions about your masculinity"; "You're an introvert"). Instead, you simply try to clarify what is unclear. Put differently, you make a guess at the feelings and content that seem to be just below the surface and check the accuracy of your understanding. Egan (1976) has noted that this level of empathy can take several forms:

Expressing what is only implied. Often a deeper understanding of another person's feelings can come from what is *not* expressed verbally. Body language, the context of the conversation and its logical implications can enhance understanding. Take a close look at what this person is saying:

> School isn't easy. Sure, I've gotten a few C's, but I keep at it. It can really be frustrating when you do your best and still don't come out on top. But I'm the first in my family to go to college. I'm pretty sure I'll get a B average this semester.

At one level this person is telling us that he sometimes gets frustrated (his emotion) over a low grade (factual content). This would be an example of primary-level accurate empathy. But let us think about the logical implications of what he is saying. School isn't easy . . . he is the first in his family to go to college . . . he's pretty sure of a good grade this semester . . . low grades frustrate him. These are the kinds of concerns a very *committed* and *determined* student might have. A response reflecting advanced-level accurate empathy might be:

Correct me if I'm wrong, but I sense you are very committed to school and determined to get through.

Summarizing. If the other person has expressed a number of feelings and concerns, it can be useful to bring them together in a summary. This helps the other person see many bits and pieces together, and perhaps gain a new perspective. Here is an example of a summarizing empathic response:

> In the last half hour you've shared a lot. Let's see if I've got it straight. You're having trouble in some classes, but have decided to work to complete school. Your relationship with your wife seems to be going sour, but you think it's time to talk to her and deal directly with problems that might arise. At work, they're beginning to add responsibilities to your job; you'll try to do a good job, but you've decided to have a talk with your supervisor.

Identifying themes. It is often helpful to look for common threads that run through what the other person is sharing with you. You might want to think of what the underlying message, or theme is. It can even be useful to imagine that the other person is telling you a short story from his or her life, and you are to come up with a thematic title. In the example we just examined, one theme might be expressed this way:

> I've been thinking about some of the things you've been saying. It's almost as if you're telling me that you are becoming more of an assertive person. You seem determined to deal with problems and state what's on your mind.

The Empathic Role

The most general way of looking at accurate empathy is in terms of the role you play. You are, of course, not playing psychologist, priest, parent, or police officer. You are a collaborative helper, working together with the other person to try to understand them better. Your empathic responses are tentative, and you invite candid reactions and corrections. Donald Meichenbaum (1985) has listed a variety of phrases and probes that convey this role.

Correct me if I am wrong, but what I hear you saying is . . .

I am not sure if I quite understood; can we go over that one more time?

I am wondering in what ways your becoming stressed in situation . . . is like your becoming stressed in situation . . . ?

On the one hand I hear you saying . . . and on the other hand I hear you saying. . . . I wonder how these two things go together.

You seem to be telling me. . . . Am I correct in assuming that . . . ?

I get the feeling that. . . . Is that the way you see it?

We have covered a lot of territory so far. Is there anything I said that troubled you?[1]

[1]Meichenbaum, D.C. (1985). *Stress Inoculation Training.* Elmsford, NY: Pergamon Press, pp. 29–30.

EXERCISE 20.1 *Understanding Yourself Empathically*

Here is a useful empathy exercise that Egan (1976) suggests. Begin by describing a stressful situation you recently encountered. Include all the specifics: what happened, who was involved, what you and the other person(s) did and said, and what you thought and felt.

Example:

My husband and I have two children, twin boys who are ten years old. Recently my husband yelled at one of the boys, Tom, for coming home late after school. This upset me. I thought it would have been better to first find out why Tom was late, and if he had no good reason, negotiate a firm policy about when he should come home. My husband simply wouldn't listen to my ideas. He seemed to feel he had all the answers. I felt really low, like I wasn't worth a thing.

Your example:

Next, imagine you are a good friend listening to your problem. Write down a good, empathic response, using the criteria introduced in this chapter. Be sure to focus on both feelings and content.

Example:

I hear your feelings of hurt. You're sad that your husband wouldn't even listen to a very important idea you had.

Your example:

EXERCISE 20.2 *Looking for Empathy*

Here is another interesting exercise Egan suggests. If you spend time listening to others, you will often find both good and bad examples of empathy. For the next few days, spend a few minutes listening to people in a variety of public settings—in the cafeteria, on the streets, on the bus or in the locker room. See if you can identify responses that are truly empathic and those that lack empathy. Try to identify why it is present or not present. When you hear a nonempathic response, think of what you might say that would be more empathic.

Stress and Life

Coping is a life skill. Like breathing, eating, and keeping fit, it is a full-time activity. In Chapters 21–23 we take a broader look at coping and work, school, and home. We examine managing our time and priorities as a coping strategy. And we conclude with the all-important challenge of taking stock of our deficiencies, and tapping our hidden resources.

21

MANAGING WORK STRESS

Target Coping Skills

- Identifying sources of stress at work
- Managing stress from work responsibilities
- Managing stress from amount of workload
- Managing stress resulting from work environment
- Identifying symptoms of burnout

Purpose

- On-the-job stress
- Stress at school
- Stress in sports
- Stress from managing family matters

Example

Rob works as a nurse in a local hospital. Although his job is difficult, he feels that much of his stress is needless. He has identified several sources of stress at the hospital: noisy, cold, foul-smelling work conditions; unclear job descriptions; and too much work. After looking at this list, it was clear that he had to talk to the supervisor and ask for help. Together, they decided to set half a day aside for a job stress workshop. In this workshop they clarified each nurse's job responsibilities. Strategies were discussed for reducing workload. Finally, they practiced giving each other helpful and constructive feedback. CUE → COPE → REWARD summary: IDENTIFICATION OF SOURCES OF STRESS → DISCUSSION WITH SUPERVISOR AND WORKSHOP → FEEDBACK AND RESOLUTION

Job-related stress is one of the hottest topics in business today. The reasons are clear. About 14 percent of the occupational diseases on workers' compensation claims appear to be stress-related. And insurance claim benefits for stress average $15,000—twice the amount for physical injury (McCarthy, 1988). An average of one million workers are absent on any given day primarily because of stress disorders (Rosh & Pelletier, 1987). In what is perhaps one of the most widely cited stress statistics, stress may well cost business over $150 billion a year in lowered productivity, absenteeism, and disability (Pelletier & Lutz, 1988).

Evidence is mounting that funding for stress management education is a good investment. The Kennecott Copper Corporation reduced sickness and accident costs by 75% when they introduced stress management courses at work (Egdahl & Walsh, 1980). The PA Medical Corporation reduced absenteeism by 14% by instituting a stress reduction program (Everly & Girdano, 1980). Further, Carol Schneider, past president of the American Biofeedback Society, has estimated that businesses can save an average of five dollars for every dollar spent on stress management (Schneider, 1987).

However, one important fact is often missed in the current explosion of interest in work stress. The very factors that contribute to stress on the job can contribute to stress in other areas of life, including: volunteer work, vacationing, managing leisure and recreation, doing household chores, organizing school activities, participating in sports, running a family, and even something as simple as setting up a car pool. In each of these areas, stress-related absenteeism, tardiness, accidents, illness, substance abuse, and reduced morale and productivity can be important concerns. What is traditionally called "occupational stress" can perhaps more appropriately be called "the stress of managing the tasks of living."

Sources of "Work Stress"

Other chapters of this book consider many factors important for understanding work stress—changes in life events, Type A behavior, lack of control, difficulty with problem-solving, negative thinking, unassertiveness, lack of relaxation skills, conflict, and inability to negotiate or to empathize. However, in this chapter we will consider factors related to the type of work one does, whether it be on the job, as a volunteer or in school. Specifically, we will consider three factors: workload, or the amount of work to be done; specific types of work responsibilities; and the work environment.

Workload

How often have you complained about being overworked? It may not surprise you that overload is one of the chief sources of work stress. When you feel you have too much work to do in too little time, you are suffering from *quantitative overload.* Quantitative overload is especially serious when you have little control over the rate at which you must complete your work (Hurrell, 1987). However, if time is not the problem but rather your lack of training or ability to do the job, you are experiencing *qualitative overload.* Finally, sometimes work *underload*, or too little work, can be stressful. Some factors that can aggravate underload are: (1) a mechanically controlled pace of work; (2) repetitiveness; (3) few demands placed on worker skills; (4) predetermined tools and techniques; (5) highly specialized tasks; and (6) little demand on worker attention (Walker & Guest, 1952).

Work Responsibilities

There are times when work is stressful even when you have adequate time, skill, and ability. The specific nature of your defined responsibilities can be a problem. We can see this in the following example:

> Marge is starting work as a social worker in a local community clinic. At first, her work involved counseling clients. This is an enjoyable task, one she expected to do at the clinic. However, over the next few months state funding for the clinic was cut back and a number of staff members had to be laid off. Marge found herself doing such secretarial work as typing reports, filing papers, and answering the phone. At times, unexpected emergencies would get in the way of her counseling duties; for example, she would have to answer the phone for her supervisor while a client was waiting. From time to time staff members from other departments would call on her to help out. In addition to such hassles, Marge found her job less secure, and the possibilities for career advancement less likely.

It is easy to see that Marge is under considerable stress. At first she knew what was expected of her. However, as funding was cut back, she found her duties less clear. Such a problem is called *role ambiguity.* It arises when one's work role, or defined responsibilities, is poorly defined. A similar problem, *role conflict*, occurs when one job duty conflicts with, or is incompatible, with another or with your personal standards. Marge found it impossible to answer the phone and see clients at the same time. She was also upset by having to do secretarial work since she was trained to be a social worker. Such problems can be made worse by *job insecurity* or *lack of opportunities for career advancement.*

Too much or too little *responsibility for others* can be an important source of job stress. Such stress can come from having to evaluate others for pay raises, promotions, or dismissal; from having to offer incentives; and from managing employee problems and shortcomings. However, not having responsibility or authority can also be stressful, especially in very demanding jobs. For example, you may have complex work to complete, and yet have to clear every action with your supervisors. Or you may be in a position to see how things go wrong and can be improved, but have little authority to make changes or even express your opinion.

Job reviews and assessments are rarely pleasant. However, the manner in which such evaluations are handled can create needless stress. Particularly destructive are unfair and arbitrary reviews in which expectations are not clearly or openly defined. In addition, criteria for evaluation may well be clear, but insufficient feedback is given, leaving you in the dark as to how well you are doing. Finally, evaluators often tend to focus on negative feedback and ignore the positive. This may not be deliberate or malicious, but a simple consequence of the way we deal with problems in our society. If something is going wrong, it has to be corrected, otherwise the problem may continue;

negative feedback is often an absolute requirement to set things right. However, when things are going well, there is no urgent need to make changes or give feedback. Unfortunately, people learn best when they receive positive feedback, and they find excessive negative feedback frustrating and demoralizing.

Work Environment

Many factors can make even the best job stressful because of poor work conditions, including: lack of physical or financial resources, noise, heat, cold, too much or too little light, odors, pollution, crowding, lack of privacy, and even desk layout. To some extent, individuals can differ in the types of environment they can tolerate. For example, one employee might tolerate the noise in an automobile factory while another may need the quiet of an executive office. People differ in their preferences for sound and light levels and need for privacy. However, most of us *habituate* to, or become insensitive to, constant environmental assaults. After a few months you may get used to living next to an airport or in a polluted city. Nonetheless, your environment can still contribute to stress-related illness, even outside of your awareness.

Burnout

Burnout is one of the long-term costs of work stress. It is typically defined in terms of three symptoms (Freudenberger, 1980; Jackson, Schwab, & Schuler, 1986; Maslach & Jackson, 1981).

1. Emotional exhaustion, or feeling drained and empty because of excessive work demands. We can see such emotional exhaustion in the following examples:
   I no longer look forward to going to work each morning.
   At the end of each day I feel totally drained and exhausted. I no longer have the energy and enthusiasm I used to.
   I just plod through each day's chores.
2. Depersonalization, or becoming insensitive, closed off, callous, cynical, or hostile towards others:
   Why can't my clients (students/customers) be more responsible?
   I find myself treating the people I work with as objects.
   I just can't get myself to care about their problems.
   My clients are just lazy and good for nothing. They'll never change.
3. Low feelings of accomplishment, or feeling frustrated and helpless because your efforts are wasted and worthless:
   Boy, I made a mistake getting into this line of work. Nothing I do makes any difference.
   I feel like my life is a waste.
   I'm really depressed and blue about my job.

Burnout appears to be particularly high in human service and helping professions (such as physicians, nurses, counselors, teachers, social workers, police). It is also prevalent in people who are highly invested in, and committed to, their work. Such people often experience a "honeymoon" of enthusiasm and optimism, only to discover later that their work does not fit their initial, high expectations.

Examples of Work Stress

As we noted earlier, it is important to note that work stress is a very broad concept. It can apply to a variety of contexts outside of places of employment. We can see this in the following examples. In the first, we have identified some of the sources of stress. In the following two, see if you can identify what creates stress.

Volunteering

Work overload

Role Ambiguity

Burnout

Roberta has volunteered to help out in a fund raising drive for her singing group. After a few weeks, she finds herself doing more than she expected. At first she answered phones, then stuffed envelopes, and then spent the weekend seeking donations from door to door. She feels like she has little time left for her family, and that this volunteer work has become a "bottomless pit." With all this work, Roberta is beginning to get cynical about volunteer work in general. She feels, "Everyone wants to volunteer, but no one wants to do the work."

Vacationing

Burt and Julia have decided to take their family on a summer vacation. Their plans are to drive across the country and see the sights. Julia has been doing the driving and has made a few mistakes. Burt starts complaining, "Why didn't you check the map before getting on the turnpike? Now we have to turn off to see where we're going. And didn't you check the oil at the last gas station? Can't you do anything right?" Later on, Burt and Julia get into an argument. Both want to drive in the morning. Burt complains, "We agreed that I would do the morning driving and you would drive in the afternoon." Julia disagrees.

Cleaning the Apartment

Bill and Bob have been college roommates for over a year. However, some problems have been brewing. Bob finally confronts Bill: "This year's lease is about up and you still haven't let me know if we will be rooming together next year. This uncertainty isn't good. I need to know what's going to happen." Bill responds that he will continue rooming with Bob. However, there are a few issues he wants to clear up: "Let's make it clear just who is responsible for the dishes, and who has to dust and vacuum. I'm feeling overburdened by all the jobs that have to get done around here. This place is just too dusty for me to feel comfortable."

Managing Work Stress

In their most general terms, the stress management techniques noted in this book can be applied to work stress. However, a few specific strategies are worth highlighting. Often what you can do depends on whether or not your coworkers and supervisors are cooperative, that is, if they are interested and willing to do something about job stress.

Strategies for a Cooperative Situation

When the people around you are willing to consider change, your assertiveness and negotiation might be enough to start the process of making the workplace less stressful. Gathering information is a useful place to begin. If your problem is role conflict or ambiguity, job insecurity, or lack of feedback on how you are doing, the Bower and Bower (1976) DESC script can help. As we noted earlier in this book, the DESC script includes four types of statements:

Describe: Describe what aspects of work are causing problems.

Express: Express what you think and feel about this problem.

Specify: Specify what specific, concrete, and realistic changes you would like.

Consequences: Spell out what will be the specific, concrete, and realistic consequences if your problem is resolved (or not resolved). That is, what are the payoffs of solving the problem, and the costs of not solving it?

Here is an application of the DESC script to a problem of role ambiguity:

Situation: You and your friends are planning a camping trip. Various camping chores have been delegated. However, you find you end up doing chores that are not yours.

Describe: "Yesterday we agreed that I would be responsible for buying food for our trip. Today, I ended up cleaning up after breakfast and lunch, which was not my responsibility."

Express: "I feel like I'm getting more than my share of chores. I don't like feeling like the one who has to do everything around here."

Specify: "We agreed that I would buy the food, and someone else would clean up after eating. I would like to keep to that agreement. If we can't, let's work out a different way of dividing up the chores, one that is fair."

Consequences: "If everyone does their fair share of work on this trip, no one will feel overburdened and we'll all have plenty of time to enjoy the trip."

In work situations, a clear statement of one's responsibilities, as well as clear feedback on how well one is doing, can do much to reduce stress. The following "Specify" statements and questions can be very useful:

"I would like you to clarify exactly what my work role is. What are my jobs, and what jobs belong to someone else?"

"I would like to know specifically what I am doing right. What do you see as my strengths?"

"What specific areas of my work need improving? It would be helpful to me if you could identify specific examples."

"I need to know just where I stand. If I continue to perform as I am performing now, what will be the consequences?"

"When can I consider my work finished? What am I expected to do, and what are the responsibilities of others?"

Sometimes, a modification of the work setting is required to reduce stress. This can be as simple as reducing noise or crowding, or altering uncomfortable temperature levels. Sometimes a restructuring of the tasks themselves can be useful. You may want to consider changes in these areas (Everly & Girdano, 1980; Girdano, Everly, & Dusek, 1990; Rosch & Pelletier, 1987).

How can I use more of my skills? A monotonous, unchanging job that does little to tap your abilities can contribute to considerable stress. Are there other jobs you can do? Can responsibilities be shared to make work more interesting and challenging?

How can I see what good my work has done? It can be stressful to be a meaningless cog in a giant machine. People like to see what impact they have had on a finished product. For example, it is frustrating for a teacher to spend long hours counseling a troubled child and never see if this work pays off later on. An assembly line worker may attach one specific part on an automobile and never see the finished product he or she helped build. It is more satisfying to have opportunities to see what you have done. In that vein, Swedish automobile workers now act as a team, each working on a single automobile from start to finish.

How can I have more say in what I do? Autonomy is having some say over what you do and when you do it. For example, in a flextime work schedule you can determine when you start and end work and when to take breaks, as long as you put in a certain number of hours a day. Autonomy can also extend to your specific job tasks. Can you acquire some control over which tasks you do at which times?

How can I know more about what's going on, and have a chance to make my views heard? In democratic, or participative management, workers have some say in how things are run. They have a chance to find out organizational policies and goals and clearly voice their opinions, make suggestions, and even participate in decisions that have to be made. This can be achieved with a simple suggestion box, or by means of meetings in which all opinions are aired.

How can I improve myself at work, and contribute to my career development? If you have concerns about your career development, take a close look at how your present work contributes to your goals. Does it require the development and practice of skills you can use later on? Are you increasing your knowledge in areas that are important to you? If you feel your job is stagnant, consider how it can be restructured to contribute to your growth.

What are the rewards and penalties for my job performance? Specifically, how will you benefit for work well done? When will you be rewarded? What will be the specific costs for mistakes or inadequate work? When will you have to pay for them? Finally, try to minimize needless punitive controls.

Strategies for the Upcooperative Situation

Let's be realistic—often there are precious few opportunities to change one's work. And quitting is not always an option. In such situations, it is important to know how to survive and avoid burnout. Once again, all of the approaches mentioned in this book can be useful. Those most frequently mentioned by job stress experts include:

Think realistically about work; try to avoid catastrophizing.

Separate your self-worth from the task you are doing. You are a good and worthwhile person, even though your job may be frustrating.

Distinguish between what you really need, and what would be nice to have. Try to avoid treating your wishes as if they were necessities.

Look for ways to meet your needs and use your untapped skills outside of work. If you need to be with people but you work alone, then seek social activities outside of work. If you have good public speaking skills and do not use them at work, consider joining clubs where you can speak out.

Treasure your relaxation and leisure time. They can help you recover from, and prevent, much work stress. You must preserve your moments of relaxation and not use them for tasks such as homework.

Nurture and use your social support networks. Spend time with your friends and family. Share your feelings and frustrations.

Finally, look for humor in frustration. Of course, "laughing it off," and "putting on a happy face" are hardly rational and useful ways to deal with stress. However, there is a time for humor. Often the impossible predicaments that life dishes out can make quite a tale of absurdity when told to someone else. Sometimes, the best way of dealing with stress is to simply stand back, look at things in perspective, and laugh.

EXERCISE 21.1 *Analyzing a Job*

In this exercise, think of a job you have had that created considerable stress. Describe this job below.

Now, using the principles discussed in this chapter, identify the main sources of job stress.

What approaches to stress management might be most appropriate for this job? Use any of the approaches discussed in this or other chapters.

What are some of the strengths and weaknesses of each of the approaches you have named?

22

MANAGING TIME

Target Coping Skills

- Setting goals and priorities
- Stopping "time wasters"
- Scheduling

Purpose

- Identification of long-term and short-term priorities
- Creation of efficient weekly and daily schedules
- Effective work plan
- Solution to "feeling rushed" or "never having enough time"

Example

Gretchen never seems to have enough time to do what she wants. Even though she always seems to be busy, things just do not get done. Once she recognized how busy she felt, she decided to construct a time management plan. Using the concepts of this chapter, she carefully identified her long-term and short-term priorities. She determined one or two "absolute must" tasks for each week. After carefully monitoring how she spends her time, she discovered a number of ways in which she thoughtlessly wastes time, including vacillating between various tasks, obsessing about what should be done, and spending needless time chatting on the phone. Her reward was to schedule one extra day off that month. CUE → COPE → REWARD summary: EXCESSIVE BUSYNESS → REARRANGEMENT OF PRIORITIES AND SCHEDULING → EXTRA DAY OFF

People often think of time as a source of stress. This is revealed in a variety of popular phrases, such as:

Time is money.
Haste makes waste.
You only go around once.
A stitch in time saves nine.
Make hay while the sun shines.
There's no time like the present.
Time flies.
Time waits for no one.
Yesterday is but a dream.

However, it is a bit misleading to think of time itself as the culprit. After all, time itself is constant and can't be altered; no matter what you do, there will still be 24 hours in a day and 12 months in a year. When people complain about time, they usually have problems like the following: too much work, conflicts between tasks, missed deadlines, feelings of being overwhelmed by trivia, and inability to do what one wants because of unfinished tasks. The key to coping with such problems involves many of the strategies presented elsewhere in this book, including identifying what to do with your time, rationally considering your goals, assertively standing up for your rights, and setting time aside for relaxation. This is time management.

Alan Lakein (1973) is often cited as a well-known expert in time management. His practical ideas can be organized into four steps.

The Four Steps of Time Management

Step 1: How Do You Spend Your Time?

Most people have only a fuzzy idea of how they specifically spend each part of the day. How do you spend your day? To answer this question, try dividing your day into half-hour segments and record what you do in each segment. For example, Bill is a college student who never seems to have enough time to do the things he wants. Here is how he recorded one day:

8:00 A.M. Wake up
8:00–8:30 Stay in bed deciding on whether to get up
8:30–9:00 Watch TV
9:00–9:30 Get dressed
9:30–10:00 Eat breakfast
10:00–10:30 Watch TV
10:30–11:00 Study
11:00–12:00 Attend class
12:00–12:30 Talk with friends
12:30–1:00 Read paper
1:00–1:30 Eat lunch

1:30–2:00 Study

2:00–2:30 Walk back to room

2:30–3:00 Get ready for practice in gym

3:00–3:30 Talk with friends on phone

3:30–4:00 Practice in gym

4:00–4:30 Walk home

4:30–5:00 Get ready for dinner

5:00–6:00 Study

6:00–7:00 Eat dinner

7:00–8:00 Talk with friends

8:00–9:00 Watch TV

9:00–10:00 Get ready for bed

10:00–10:30 Study

10:30–11:00 Watch TV

11:00–11:30 Talk with friends

Once you have charted a day, decide what major activities you engage in. Group together activities that are similar (such as reading the paper and watching TV, or eating and preparing meals). Bill discovered he engaged in the following:

Studying

Attending class

Eating

Socializing

Solitary recreation

Getting in/out of bed; getting dressed

Preparing for and practicing in gym

Traveling

Now, divide your day into three segments: morning to 12 noon; 12 noon to 6 PM; 6 PM to bedtime. Using your activity list, indicate how many hours are spent on each activity for each time period. Here is Bill's analysis:

Morning–12:00 Noon

Hours	Activity
½	Studying
1	Attending class
½	Eating
0	Socializing
1	Solitary recreation
1	Getting ready for bed; getting dressed
0	Preparing for and practicing in gym
0	Traveling

12:00 Noon–6:00 p.m.

Hours	Activity
1½	Studying
0	Attending class
1	Eating
1	Socializing
½	Solitary recreation
0	Getting ready for bed; getting dressed
1	Preparing for and practicing in gym
1	Traveling

6:00 p.m.–Bedtime

Hours	Activity
½	Studying
0	Attending class
1	Eating
1½	Socializing
1½	Solitary recreation
1	Getting ready for bed; getting dressed
0	Preparing for and practicing in gym
0	Traveling

Now, complete an overall tally of your day's activities. How many hours do you spend on each? Here is Bill's summary:

Summary

Hours	Activity
2½	Studying
1	Attending class
2½	Eating
2½	Socializing
3	Solitary recreation
1½	Getting ready for bed; getting dressed
1	Preparing for and practicing in gym
1	Traveling

After examining his summary, Bill was surprised how much time he spent on solitary recreation, getting ready for bed and getting dressed. Perhaps some of your activities, like Bill's, could be cut back or done more efficiently. However, for the time being, put your chart aside. We will return to it later.

Step 2: What Are Your Long-Term Goals and Priorities?

Time management begins with a bit of soul-searching. What are your goals in life? First consider your lifetime goals. What really matters to you? In considering your goals, think about what you truly value in life. Here are some values many people consider important:

Satisfying family life

Beauty

Spirituality and "meaning of life"

Financial success

Fame and recognition

Discovery

Adventure

Artistic creation and expression

Personal effectiveness

Power

Love

What are your lifetime goals? What will make you satisfied and contented when you retire? Next, consider your five-year goals. These are relatively long-term objectives which you can envision at this time. Finally, what are your objectives for the next three to six months? In considering this exercise, it is important to stand back from yourself and take an objective stance. How might a trusted friend advise you about your various goals? Here are the goals Bill has considered:

Life-time goals

To have a family

To have a good job

To keep healthy

Five-year goals

To successfully complete college

To get my first job

To have a steady girlfriend, and maybe get married

Six-month goals

To successfully complete one year of college

To move out of the dormitory and find an apartment on my own (or with a roommate)

To earn enough money to pay for another year of college

Considering your long-term goals, which are most important? Which are less important? Which should you start considering today? Which can be put off for a time? Bill has decided that his immediate priority is to get through school with good grades. Without this, he will not be able to get a good job, or comfortably support a family—his other long-term goals.

Now consider your main goal, one you can start working on right away. Break this into concrete, specific, and realistic steps. Brainstorm possible courses of action (Chapter 4). What specific things will you have to do to obtain your goal? Bill decided his main goal was figuring out how to complete one year of college. Here is his analysis:

To successfully complete one year of college

Get enough money to pay my way

Find a part-time job

Look for a long-term job

Take courses that will develop job skills

Make acquaintances who can find me work

Do volunteer work that might prepare me for a job

Take reasonable courses

Seek advice from counselors

Ask my friends about what courses to take

Study enough to get good grades

Set aside enough time to study

Use a rational study and review plan

Step 3: What Are Your Goals and Priorities for Today and for This Week?

Now, you need to make some decisions about what to do. Consider your short-term priorities for today and for this week. Lakein suggests developing "top drawer," "middle drawer," "bottom drawer," and "waste basket" priorities. Top drawer priorities are your most important tasks today and this week. Imagine you earn 80% of your rewards from only 20% of your activities. What would the 20% activities include? In the middle drawer, include activities you would like to do today and this week. However, they are activities that could be put off if absolutely necessary. Finally, bottom drawer priorities include tasks that you will do only when you have finished your top and middle drawer tasks. These are activities that do not have to be done with any urgency. Finally, "waste basket" priorities are activities that simply are a waste of time. They do not have to be completed at all, ever. Bill decided to prioritize his activities for one week and then one day. Looking at his chart, here is his analysis:

THIS WEEK

Top Drawer

Read first three chapters in my history text.

Select a topic for my term paper.

Ask Alice out for a date.

Eat and sleep.

Middle Drawer

Read Chapter 4 for next week, if I have time.

Practice in the gym.

Spend some time with my friends.

Read the paper.

Bottom Drawer

Watch TV.

Waste Basket

Sit around.

TODAY

Top Drawer

Read and outline Chapter 1.

Phone Alice. Talk with her no more than an hour.

Middle Drawer

Practice in gym.

Read the paper.

Bottom Drawer

Watch TV.

Talk with my friends (I can do that tomorrow).

Waste Basket

Sit around.

Step 4: What Is the Best Way to Schedule Your Activities?

Now go back to your schedule. This time, write in those activities that make the most sense in terms of your goals. However, it is important to be realistic. Schedule in periodic times for relaxation and rewarding activities. Remember those obligations over which you have little control (such as traveling, sleeping and eating).

Pick the best time to do your important activities. Lakein suggests thinking in terms of internal and external prime time. Internal prime time is when you do your best private work (studying, writing reports and letters and organizing plans). External prime time is when external resources are most available (when the library is least crowded; when your boss is there to answer questions, when your girlfriend is most likely to be available for a date).

Once again, in making your schedule remember to include reasonable "chunks" of activities, those you are likely to complete and feel good about in the time allotted. First take a look at your original schedule summary. Which activities are receiving too much or too little time? What part of the day needs the greatest change? Once you have considered these issues, write another summary schedule, and a specific schedule. Here is Bill's general schedule for today:

8:00 A.M.	Wake up
8:00–8:30	Get dressed
8:30–9:00	Eat breakfast
9:00–9:30	Study Chapter 1. (This is "prime time" because my roommate's in class and can't bother me)
9:30–10:00	Study Chapter 1
10:00–10:30	Read paper if finished with study; otherwise continue studying
10:30–11:00	Reward myself by watching TV
11:00–12:00	Attend class
12:00–1:00	Eat lunch
1:00–1:30	Study and review Chapter 1 (I'll study in the library. This is prime time because few people are there)
1:30–2:00	Study
2:00–2:30	Study
2:30–3:00	If finished with study, go to room to get ready for gym
3:00–3:30	Practice in gym
3:30–4:00	Practice in gym
4:00–4:30	Go back to room
4:30–5:30	Call Alice (This is "prime time" because I know she's home at this hour and isn't doing anything)
5:30–6:00	Get ready for dinner
6:00–7:00	Eat dinner

7:00–8:00	Watch TV
8:00–9:00	Talk with friends
9:00–11:00	Study
11:00–11:30	Get ready for bed

Procrastination

Even the best schedule is worthless if it does not lead to action. Dealing with procrastination is an important side of time management. We will consider two general strategies: combating procrastinating thoughts and behaviors.

Procrastinating Thoughts

A variety of irrational and self-defeating beliefs can interfere with completing a desired plan. Here are a few:

I shouldn't try because I might not fully succeed.

I shouldn't try because I'm not sure I can deal with success.

I must "feel motivated" before I do anything.

I won't attempt something unless I can be perfect at it.

I can achieve any goal without setback or frustration.

David Burns (1989) has a clever approach for dealing with procrastinating thoughts. He calls it the "TIC-TOC Technique." It's very simple. First identify your Task-Interfering Cognitions (your "TICs"). They might be any of the ones we have just mentioned. Then think them through. How do they represent negative thinking? Then, replace your thoughts with Task-Oriented Cognitions ("TOCs"). In the following example, you might identify the following as a TIC:

"I shouldn't try because I might not fully succeed."

How is this irrational or self-defeating? Well, often half a loaf is better than none at all. There are many times in life we can't get everything we want. And success may take time. A replacement TOC might be:

"I might as well try; I'm fairly sure I'll succeed at least in part."

What TOCs can you think of for the remaining self-defeating and irrational thoughts we have mentioned?

Procrastinating Behavior

There are times when nonassertive and aggressive behavior can lead to procrastination. Nonassertive people often tend to agree to do things they do not really want to do. As a result, they have less time for themselves. Some nonassertive people express their irritation with others by delaying tasks or taking longer than necessary to finish work. Sometimes procrastination can turn into something of a power struggle, with the nonassertive person procrastinating in response to perceived unreasonable demands. When lack of assertiveness appears to be the source of procrastination, you might consider the principles of assertiveness discussed earlier in this book.

Time Management Tactics

It is easy to get stuck when developing and staying with a schedule. Popular "how to do it" books on stress management often offer extensive menus of advice on time management (Davis, Eshelman, & McKay, 1988; Grasha, 1983; & Greenberg, 1990). Here are a few of the more useful ideas frequently mentioned:

Say No and Set Limits

Learn to say no to those who place demands on you that keep you from finishing top drawer tasks. It is often useful to plan beforehand how you will handle interruptions. You might decide to say, "I'm sorry, I'm involved with something very important now. Can I talk with you later?" Another strategy is to simply state your limits, like this: "I'm really busy now and can only talk for about five minutes. Is that enough time?"

Plan Ahead for Saboteurs

The best of plans can be easily sabotaged. Someone may want to chat with you about the ballgame. Another person has a problem and seems upset. Think ahead what your saboteurs may do and plan ahead what your response will be.

Delegate

Do you absolutely have to do everything on your "to do" list? If possible, see if you can delegate middle and bottom drawer activities to someone else.

See It Through

Select one task from your top drawer and see it through to completion. Many people waste time by "nibbling" at a task, that is, doing a little bit, and then doing something else. Others obsess and return again and again to a job that has been completed. Simply finish your task and then put it away.

Remove Distractions

People who have trouble sticking with their schedules and priorities often find themselves inadvertently doing "waste basket" activities. This is more likely to happen if there are cues in your environment to distract you. Such cues might include magazines, photographs of family, unfinished letters or open doors. One good time management strategy is to remove potential distractions.

Build in "Time Buffers"

Even the best of plans can run into problems. In your schedule, build in special times which you can use to complete unfinished business or unforeseen problems. Such periods can be called "time buffers" and can increase the likelihood of your successfully completing your schedule.

Pace Yourself

Stoyva (Stoyva & Anderson, 1982) has suggested that successful copers often pace themselves throughout the day. Rather than spend all day on a single job, you should alternate your activities between work that is demanding and work that is easy.

Schedule Rewards for Completing Tasks

People with poor time management habits often fail to see the importance of carefully scheduling rewards for completing tasks. They often hold the myth that finishing a task should be its own reward. This is not how the real world operates. We are more likely to continue behaviors that are rewarded and to forget behaviors that are not rewarded. This principle works for teaching a dog new tricks and is just as valid when we teach ourselves to manage our time.

Set Aside Personal Time—And Honor It Unless you are determined to become a workaholic, it is important to reserve special times for yourself. These times should be inviolable periods for rest and fun. Use them to read, look out of a window or listen to the radio.

Remember: Time Spent Planning Is Time Invested Many people have the mistaken notion that the best way to finish a complex job is to plunge into it until it is finished. They feel that spending time developing a schedule is actually wasting time. In fact, by developing a sensible time management plan you are investing minutes that may pay off in hours saved.

EXERCISE 22.1 *Your Priorities*

Using the principles discussed in this chapter, list your lifetime, five-year, and six-month goals. Rank each according to their importance.

Lifetime goals (ranked)

Five-year goals (ranked)

Six-month goals (ranked)

EXERCISE 22.2 *Analyzing a Goal*

Select what for you is a main goal (from your goals listed in EXERCISE 22.1), a goal you can begin working on right away. List it here:

Now, list the subgoals and activities needed to achieve this goal:

EXERCISE 22.3 *Your Schedule*

Using the principles discussed in this chapter, construct a realistic schedule for your next work (or school) day. Complete each of the four steps.

EXERCISE 22.4 *Your Time Wasters*

Take a look at the time management tactics discussed in this chapter. Which do you use? Which should you use more? Can you think of any additional tactics for limiting time wasters?

EXERCISE 22.5 *Cues and Consequences*

Time management involves a variety of specific goals and tasks. Each can be treated as a potential source of stress and a potential coping strategy. In this exercise, identify which time management skill is a problem for you. What are the costs of your time management problem? What are reasonable cues and early warning signs? Next, select an appropriate coping strategy, its cue, and its reward.

23

AFFIRMING YOUR RESOURCES

Target Coping Skills

- Identifying positive outcomes from a stressful situation
- Changing helplessness to optimism and resourcefulness
- Creatively generating solutions

Purpose

- Most stress situations, especially those that seem particularly difficult

Example

Francine is single and has just been laid off from a job she has held for fifteen years. She feels helpless and overwhelmed. Applying the strategies in this chapter, she first talked to a counselor to share her feelings of fear and anxiety. In addition she tentatively began the first steps towards building a new life. Living one day at a time, she focused on simple tasks. Gradually Francine examined what general resources had been depleted through the years, and concluded that she had sunk into a rut in her job and had not developed many contacts or work-related skills. She acknowledged what resources she had, such as her ability to type, read and understand complex material, and answer the phone. Looking at the balance of her depleted and existing resources, she developed an action plan to build up her work resources. She took herself out to dinner to reward herself for this careful planning. CUE → COPE → REWARD summary: HELPLESS AND OVERWHELMED FEELING → ANALYSIS OF DEPLETED RESOURCES/IDENTIFICATION OF ACTION PLAN TO STRENGTHEN RESOURCES → DINNER

Under stress, we often feel helpless. Yet people have many resources to draw from, even in the worst of circumstances. These can be divided into three categories: personal resources, productivity resources, and partnership resources (Cramer, 1990). In this chapter we examine a simple system for looking at these resources—our personal strengths and weaknesses—and using stress as a trigger for growth.

Personal resources are the strengths you have within you—your physical capacities and mental strengths, as well as your values and beliefs. *Partnership resources* refer to your relationships—your friends, lovers, spouse, and family. A *productivity resource* is related to your ability to do something productive, or to take effective action whether it be at work, school, sports, or even a hobby. When you are feeling overwhelmed by stress, it can be useful to determine if any one of these resources is being depleted (Cramer, 1990):

Personal Resources.

- Positive attitude
- Happy feelings
- Physical stamina
- Creativity
- Flexibility
- Feelings of optimism and being in control
- Ability to concentrate
- Energy
- Decisiveness
- Health
- Ability to feel love and express oneself
- Spiritual groundedness
- A sense of commitment to something "larger than oneself"

Partnership Resources.

- Social supports
- Friends you can count on
- Family you can count on
- Relatives you can count on
- Spouse or lover you can count on
- Someone you can confide in
- Ability to reach out to others
- People who love and support you
- People you can rely on for emotional support, help, information, and companionship

Productivity Resources.

- A sense of direction
- Feeling of purpose
- Clear goals
- Clear priorities
- Sense of meaning from work
- Recognition for your contributions
- Rewarding work
- Challenging rather than threatening work and activities

- Opportunities to exercise your talents
- Sense that you are helping others

Kathryn Cramer (1990) has offered a useful set of coping strategies that involve affirming these resources. (In general, they place considerable importance on getting in touch with feelings of hurt and pain. I believe this is important, but perhaps that can best be accomplished with the assistance of a trained mental health professional as part of your coping team.) Cramer outlines her affirming suggestions according to four stages of a stressful encounter: challenge, exploration, invention, and transformation. In terms of our CUE → COPE → COSTS/BENEFITS, we can view these steps as an elaboration of "COPE":

CUE

↓

Challenge, Exploration, Invention, Transformation

↓

COSTS/BENEFITS

Challenge

Once you have calmed your initial feelings of being upset over a stress situation (by talking them through with a counselor or relaxing) you can begin to take calm and cool-headed steps towards transforming the threat into a challenge. One simple strategy is constructive self-talk.

Can You Muster Up "Just Enuff"? When we evaluate our resources under stress, we often feel we are helpless. We feel confused, overwhelmed, and frustrated. As Cramer puts it, we feel we do not have enough of what it takes, whether it be energy, intelligence, strength, or creativity. Of course, such self-talk may well be true; we may not have enough resources to obtain all that we would like. However, such appraisals are simply not useful, no matter how well they fit our feelings. More constructive self-talk, as Cramer somewhat cutely puts it, is, "At least I have *just enuff.*" For example:

I have "just enuff" strength to get past the next three hours.

I have "just enuff" energy to study three more pages.

I have "just enuff" courage to talk to one more person at this party.

Note that in each instance we are affirming the resources we do have—not some ideal traits we feel we should have to reach some ideal goal. The value of this simple exercise is to turn away from thinking pessimistically to thinking optimistically. It is a small, but important change.

What Bothers You About This Stressful Situation? As I mentioned earlier, central to this system of affirming resources is an openness to feelings. This may be done best with the help of a professional counselor. However, even some recognition of how a situation is painful or frustrating can be a useful departure for the next step. Some expressions of distress include:

I have lost someone very important to me and I feel alone.

My job has grown so complex that I feel inferior.

My grade on this exam was so low, I don't know what to do.

What Are Your Opportunities? What Are the Possibilities? This exercise is a useful exercise of the imagination. In light of the pain you have just acknowledged, what good could possibly come? What opportunities are there to learn, grow, and change? At this point, turn to the three resources—personal, partnership, and productivity. For example:

I have lost someone, . . .

- I can at least be thankful for the wonderful friends I have had in the past (personal resource).
- This gives me an opportunity to strengthen my friendships (partnership resource).
- I feel a determination to do something about reviewing my life (productivity resource).

What If I Were to . . . ? After considering the possibilities, fantasize about actually taking action. Start your fantasy with the phrase, "In light of my opportunities, what if I were to ______?"

Opportunity	**What If I Were to . . . ?**
Be thankful for past friendships.	Call up a few old friends I haven't talked to for some time.
Strengthen current friendships	Ask a few existing friends out to dinner
Do something about reviewing my life	Sit down and list my priorities for this year

Often this exercise in itself is enough to prompt change. However, with serious crises, it is not unusual for more work to be done. It is OK to treat the whole challenge phase as preparation. In terms of this book, challenge can be seen as a cue for another coping sequence—tentative exploration of your options.

Exploration

Often one begins exploration by temporarily forgetting about the pain and frustration of a stressful event. This can help you along.

The next step is to explore the status of your resources. Think about personal, partnership, and productivity resources. Which do you have left? Which are depleted? And, most important, what channels of support might be available for you to restore the resources that have been depleted?

Existing Resources	**Depleted Resources**	**Channels for Restoring Resources**
Ability to socialize and make friends	Lack of "close" intimate relationships	Friends
		Work colleagues
		Relatives
		New acquaintances

Once you have identified channels for possibly restoring your resources, you have created another cue for yet another coping sequence.

Invention How will you access the channels you have identified for restoring your resources? The process of invention involves brainstorming goals and subgoals, and then selecting which you wish to try. We can see this as follows:

Channels for Restoring Resources	Goals	Subgoals
Friends	To nurture more meaningful friendships	To call up my best friend at least three times a week
		To ask two friends over for dinner this week
		To talk with my best friends about my plans for college, and get their feedback
New acquaintances	To "break the ice" and open doors for new relationships	To attend one party every other week
		To introduce myself to at least three strangers at each party
		To find out from one stranger our common interests

Selecting a goal and subgoals is your cue for a final coping sequence—transformation.

Transformation In time, coping skills become transformed into new ways of looking at and acting in the world. Such changes take time and do not result from completing a few exercises. However, once you have spelled out your goals and subgoals and have acted on them, you can sit back and reflect. What has actually happened? What worked and what did not? What resources have you begun to restore? Which still remain unrestored? What new resources have you discovered? What new deficiencies have you discovered?

Taken together, the steps we have considered outline an optimistic perspective on life. It is one that recognizes frustrations, irritations and pains. But it goes on and diligently identifies what good can come out of a stressful situation. It is an approach that attempts to replace the confusion and helplessness many feel under stress with an empowering sense of order. One can say "Yes, there may be things I can do. But I don't have to solve everything at once—just as much as I can handle. Let the future take care of itself." It is also a way of facing that future, and exploring the ever-expanding opportunities it can yield.

EXERCISE 23.1 *"I Have Just 'Enuff"*

What is your stress situation?

How is it frustrating, confusing, or overwhelming?

Right now, how would you answer this question?

I have just "enuff" . . . (describe resource)

to achieve . . . (describe goal)

EXERCISE 23.2 *Opportunities from Stress*

Now step back and with your imagination think of what opportunities might possibly be presented by this stressful situation. Consider the hypothetical question, "What if I were to . . . ?"

Opportunities	What if I were to . . . ?

EXERCISE 23.3 *Channels for Restoring Resources*

Take a look at which resources you possess and which have been depleted. Brainstorm various channels for depleting those that have been depleted.

Existing Resources	Depleted Resources	Possible Channels for Restoring Resources

EXERCISE 23.4 *Goals and Subgoals for Restoring Resources*

Consider what general channels may exist for restoring your depleted resources. What goals and subgoals can you think of?

Depleted Resource	Channel	Goals	Subgoals

Special Problems

In the real world, even the best coping strategies can go wrong. One of the most important coping skills is dealing with special problems that can arise. In Chapters 24–28 we consider negative and interfering behaviors, relapse prevention, desensitization and stress inoculation, defense, and pain.

24

CONTROLLING NEGATIVE BEHAVIORS

Target Coping Skills

- Reducing reminder cues for negative behaviors
- Reducing negative behaviors through selective punishment

Purpose

- Prevention of overeating
- Control of drinking
- Prevention of substance abuse
- Cessation of smoking
- Increase in exercise
- Any behavior that gets in the way of a reasonable coping plan

Example

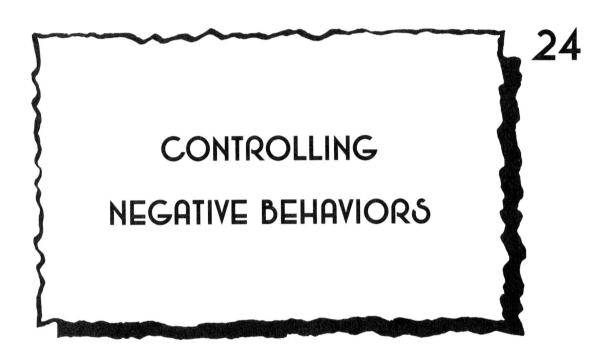

Gary is seriously out of shape, and this contributes to a general lack of energy for dealing with stressful problems. He has an exercise plan, but frequently sabotages it by snacking at 4:00 P.M., the very time he should exercise. He decides on a behavior-change plan that involves punishing snacking behavior (by depriving himself of dessert at dinner), and rewarding himself for exercise (by letting himself have dessert). CUE → COPE → REWARD summaries: 4:00 P.M. → SNACK → PUNISHMENT OF NO DESSERT and 4:00 P.M. → EXERCISE → DESSERT

People have a way of creating problems for themselves. Just about everyone has had the experience of doing or thinking something that gets in the way of coping. Such negative, interfering habits can include a variety of unhealthy behaviors that sap strength, contribute to fatigue, and thereby interfere with coping:

Not getting enough sleep

Overeating

Abusing alcohol

Abusing drugs

Smoking cigarettes

Abusing prescription medications

Avoiding exercise

Negative behaviors can include a variety of self-destructive or stress-avoiding thoughts and actions, including:

Making excuses for procrastinating

Catastrophizing or exaggerating the seriousness of stress

Behaving passively when assertive action is appropriate

Not sticking to schedules

Engaging in some stress-producing activity instead of a daily relaxation routine

In fact, just about every coping skill considered in this book can be blocked by a negative behavior, as seen below:

Coping Skill (and Chapter)	**Negative, Interfering Behavior**
Studying this chapter by using the PARET method (Introduction)	Forgetting to do the PARET method, and instead just reading the chapter twice and putting it aside
Engaging in a daily physical or mental relaxation exercise to reduce stress (Chapters 10–14)	Using your relaxation period to watch TV
Identifying when you are thinking about a stressful situation in such a way that exaggerates the consequences and creates needless tension (Chapter 6)	Avoiding a stressful situation after you have exaggerated its seriousness
Replacing a negative, catastrophizing thought, "This is the end of the world," with a more realistic thought, "This is a frustration, but I can deal with it." (Chapter 7)	Feeling sorry for yourself after thinking a negative, catastrophizing thought: "The end of the world . . . what a terrible fix I am in!"

Identifying how a stressful situation can indeed be an opportunity to grow and develop new skills (Chapter 9)	Giving up and feeling hopeless after a stressful situation
Getting to know new people by asking open-ended questions that permit them to talk about themselves (Chapter 15)	Following up an open-ended question by a closed-ended, "yes-no" question: "Did you see the news on TV tonight?"
Using the DESC script method to make an important request from others; remembering that step "E" involves sharing your emotions or feelings that are involved (Chapter 16)	Making an important request, but instead of sharing your feelings about it, you say, "It would be nice if you do what I am requesting. But, it's not that important. Don't put yourself out."
Recognizing when you are likely to respond to a provocation with inappropriate anger, and then reminding yourself to "Take it easy. One step at a time. They are only human." (Chapter 17)	Working yourself up in a provocative situation by thinking, "I'm the only one who matters. Who does the other person think she is, anyway?"
Attempting to reduce another person's emotionality by focusing on the concrete facts of their criticism (Chapter 18)	Getting angry and emotional following criticism from another person and calling them names
Negotiating a work change with your boss by first clearly thinking through your most important priorities (Chapter 19)	Failing to prepare before negotiation with your boss; worrying about what your boss might demand
Responding emphatically to a friend who is upset and angry over his grade (Chapter 20)	Trying to help your angry and upset friend by giving judgmental advice, "Don't be angry. You're really a smart person."
Telling your boss that his form of negative feedback is demoralizing, and not particularly productive; asking for both negative and positive feedback (Chapter 21)	Complaining to your co-worker about "that negative supervisor"
Attempting a time-management plan by identifying two "top drawer" activities; upon finishing these, you let yourself go onto tasks that are less important (Chapter 22)	Letting yourself be distracted by a colleague who starts to talk about an unimportant issue just as you are starting your first high-priority activity; getting caught up in others' problems

Unfortunately, many people react to such negative behaviors by accusing themselves of not having enough will-power, moral strength, or ability to concentrate. They tend to see one setback as a global coping failure. Of course, the result of such global self-condemnations is often feelings of helplessness and surrender. But, as we saw in Chapter 3, it is important to identify goals that are concrete, specific, and realistic—goals that work and make sense. Getting will-power, moral strength, and concentration are frankly vague, general, and unrealistic goals that are poorly defined.

We will see how the 1→2→3 COPE system (Chapter 4) can be used to modify such negative behaviors. Specifically, we will look at steps 1 and 3, antecedent cues and costs/benefits. Our goal will be examine how to control cues as well as costs/benefits to change our behavior. The ideas in this chapter have been suggested by one of the major experts in self control, Fred Kanfer (Kanfer & Gaelick-Buys, 1991).

Cue Control

One of my nieces one used to suck her thumb. My sister solved the problem very easily by having her wear mittens. In a simple way, she used the principle of cue control to limit a negative behavior—she simply hid the reminder thumb in a mitten. As we saw in Chapter 3, many behaviors are preceded by cues. Cues are more than just unpleasant reminders that stress is about to build; they can also be unfortunate suggestions to engage in negative behavior. Bottles of liquor in the house can suggest drinking to the alcoholic; opened boxes of cigarettes can be a suggestion to the smoker who has quit. *Cue control* involves modifying suggestion cues so that they are less likely to lead to negative behaviors.

Sometimes this can involve altering the physical or social environment. You might:

- Hide food to limit snacking
- Leave credit cards at home to reduce the temptation of spending
- Avoid visiting relatives that stir up unpleasant memories
- Find an environment free from distraction for studying or practicing relaxation
- Give your cigarettes to a friend, so that it becomes more difficult (and embarrassing) for you to smoke
- Socialize with friends who are calorie counters, exercisers, or nonsmokers

There are times when it is difficult to completely eliminate cues that suggest negative behaviors. However, it can be useful to reduce the number of cues linked to the behavior. In other words, train yourself to limit your negative behavior to certain prespecified times and places. Doing this at least gives you some control over your undesired behavior. Some suggestions for doing this include:

- Overeaters might eat only in the dining room or in the presence of others.
- Insomniacs can rid the bedroom of cues for wakefulness (such as the reading chair, television, radio and stereo).
- Students can eliminate incompatible distractions from the study area. They should not sleep, eat, watch TV or use the phone in these places.

Finally, our bodies can provide cues for negative behavior. Obviously, an empty stomach can suggest eating to the overeater, and thirst can suggest drinking to the alcoholic. In addition, anxiety sensations can suggest negative coping behaviors. At times it is possible to reduce such physiological reminders:

- The overeater can fill up with high-bulk, low-calorie foods.
- The alcoholic can drink plenty of water before a party.
- Anyone can learn to effectively reduce the intensity of bodily stress cues through relaxation.

Costs/Benefits Control

If you anticipate negative interfering behaviors, plan to follow them with an adverse consequence or punishment, and then continue with our coping plan. Punish the undesired behavior, and then proceed with your desired behavior and reward. This can be seen in the following example:

> George is a heavy smoker. His smoking is a negative behavior that interferes with coping. For instance, George has difficulty talking to his professors, especially after they return tests and papers. Instead, he typically lights up a cigarette and leaves.

In this example, the professor returning a paper is a cue for lighting up a cigarette. George might think no! and gently pinch himself after the urge to smoke, and then make an appointment with the professor to discuss the paper. He could in effect, combine a punishment plan for reducing a negative behavior with a reward plan for learning a new form of coping:

PUNISHMENT PLAN	REWARD PLAN
Professor hands back paper	Professor hands back paper
↓	↓
George lights up cigarette	George makes appointment
↓	↓
PUNISHMENT	REWARD

COMBINED PUNISHMENT AND REWARD PLAN

Professor hands back paper

↓

George lights up cigarette

↓

Punishment

↓

George makes appointment

↓

Reward

A wide range of stimuli can be used as punishments, including:

- Giving up a desired reward
- Leaving a satisfying situation (leaving a party if you act nonassertively)
- Giving up free time
- Agreeing to pay a certain amount of money for every negative behavior (giving a dollar to a charity after every smoke)
- Exclaiming Stop! (verbally or mentally)
- Inflicting a mild painful stimulus (snapping a rubber band worn on the wrist)
- Engaging in a disgusting, aversive fantasy (make sure it is not rewarding!) after your undesired behavior

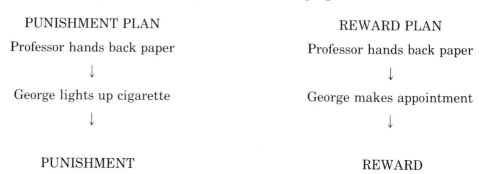

It is important to be careful in using punishments. Often their effects are only temporary. Apply punishment immediately after your negative behavior. Follow punishment with an attempt at coping, followed in turn by an appropriate review and reward. And avoid incorporating irrational or unproductive negative thinking such as awfulizing, self-blaming, or catastrophizing.

Finally, it is important to remember the power of rewards. When reducing cues to negative behavior, or following negative behavior with punishment, be sure you are also rewarding a positive replacement behavior. People often forget this. Many have the somewhat moralistic notion that, "Good behavior should come naturally," or that giving oneself a reward is somehow an indulgence. In fact, rewards strengthen behavior. Give yourself plenty of incentive to change. Practice rewarding desired behavior before actually setting up a reward plan. For more details on rewards, see Chapter 5.

EXERCISE 24.1 *Identifying Negative Behaviors*

Select a coping skill you are trying to develop. Identify a possible negative, interfering behavior. First, describe this behavior in concrete and specific terms. What are the costs of this behavior? How does it interfere with coping?

Next, what are the cues for this behavior?

Are there any ways you can modify the cues that are linked to this behavior?

What punishment can you think of to follow this behavior?

What is your coping alternative and its reward?

25

PREVENTING RELAPSE

Target Coping Skills

- Identifying "high risk" stress situations in which you might fail to use a coping strategy
- Planning a "come-back" and "fall-back" coping strategy when your coping attempts do not work

Purpose

- Any potential coping failure

Example

Lisa is trying to learn to manage her time more effectively. She has learned to create a reasonable schedule, but is afraid she will resort to her old inefficient and haphazard way of getting things done. She decides to use as her relapse cue the recognition, "Oh no, I've failed my schedule." She practices a come-back strategy that involves "schedule damage control." She takes a new look at her schedule and identifies what time has been lost, and at what time it is reasonable to resume her scheduled activities. Then, she takes a deep breath, and reassures herself, "Fine. I'm getting practice at coming back to my schedule." CUE → COPE → REWARD Summary: RECOGNITION OF FAILURE → SCHEDULE REVIEW + RESUMPTION → "FINE, I'M GETTING PRACTICE" REASSURANCE

It is quite possible that your best coping efforts may run into unexpected problems. You may get "cold feet," forget your plans or run into unanticipated obstacles. This is called relapse, and an important part of coping is anticipating and planning for setbacks through *relapse prevention*.

The key point of relapse prevention is not to give up. Relapse is often a cue for thinking such helpless thoughts as:

I'll never learn to do this.

One setback, and I'm a complete failure.

I must just be a weak person. I give up.

However, such thinking is not very helpful. Instead, it can be more useful to plan ahead for relapse.

Let us return to our college student from previous chapters. George received a low grade on an exam and wanted to speak with his professor about it. His CUE → COPE → REWARD strategy involved:

I receive my low grade. (CUE)

↓

I make an appointment with the secretary
to see the professor. (COPE)

↓

I treat myself to some ice cream. (REWARD)

(Well, here is what actually happened. Notice the relapse.)

I received my low grade. (CUE)

↓

I started to make an appointment, but got cold feet.

↓

I started thinking, "What will people think when
they see my name on the appointment sheet?"

↓

Without thinking, I walked away. (RELAPSE)

In thinking about future stressful appointments he might have to make, George decided on a number of backup strategies for dealing with relapse.

> Whenever I start thinking, "What will people think?" I'll respond by taking a deep breath and thinking, "It doesn't really matter what people think. My appointment is important." And if I start to walk away, I'll stop and think, "Walking away solves nothing. Turn around, take one step at a time, and just make the appointment." I will then make the appointment. Then I will reward myself.

Notice that George very creatively turned each relapse into a cue for what might be called a come-back strategy. In fact, the formula for all relapse prevention turns our coping formula of Chapter 5:

CUE → COPE → REWARD

Into

CUE → COMEBACK → REWARD or, if you wish,

RELAPSE → COMEBACK → REWARD

In the remainder of this chapter, we will examine a variety of powerful strategies for planning relapse comebacks.

Setbacks and Comebacks

Donald Meichenbaum (1985) has thought of a number of useful ways of getting back on track after a setback. His approach first involves dividing a stress situation into phases, for example: pre-stress, mid-stress, and post-stress. By the way, this can be valuable since many people tend to include too much in their stress problem situations. For example, Norma first described the following stress problem to her coping team:

> Today I had to write that stupid report. It was bugging me for hours. Even when I was doing something else, like answering the phone or writing letters, I worried about what I should put in the report. I wondered if I would include everything that had to be said. By the time this afternoon rolled around, I got to the report. I opened my books and started writing. Suddenly, I went blank. My heart started beating hard and I couldn't think of what to say. I put my report down, and started again a few times. Eventually I muddled through. By evening, I was finished. But the report still worries me. Why did I take so long? What's my problem?

Actually there are at least three stress situations described here, all related to writing the report. First is the period of time before writing the report. Norma worries about it even when she tries to do something else. Then comes the actually writing of the report. Norma "goes blank" and gets upset. The third situation is after the report is done. Here, the stress involves worrying about the work that has been done.

These phases can be put more formally. In any stress situation, the pre-stress phase refers to any period of time before the onset of the main event of concern. This can be months, weeks, or days. Here you are more likely to be preoccupied with feelings of anticipation concerning the future stress event. This is the time to emphasize planning and preparation. In mid-stress, the stress event is actually taking place. Finally, in the post-stress phase, the stress situation is over. However, some important things can still happen. You can put yourself down needlessly for failure, creating more stress. You can fail to recognize and nurture budding successes. And you may unproductively "replay" the stress situation in your mind.

Here are some examples of the three phases of stress:

Taking an Exam

Pre-Stress: I start studying one week before the exam. Stress builds until the day of the exam.
Mid-Stress: I am actually taking the exam.
Post-Stress: The exam is over. I think about what I did.

Attending a New Class

Pre-Stress: The week before the class begins, I get the books and think about what will be covered.
Mid-Stress: Class begins. I sit down. The instructor begins explaining class objectives.
Post-Stress: The first session is over. I walk out of class. What a relief!

Protesting an Incorrect Billing

Pre-Stress: I think about what I will say when I talk to my salesperson.
Mid-Stress: I walk up to the salesperson and protest the bill.
Post-Stress: There, I've protested. I walk away and review what I did right and wrong.

The value of breaking a stress situation down into phases is that it forces us to clarify our cues, goals, and as we shall see later, the possibility for relapse. Each phase has its own cues and goals, as we can see on the following list:[1]

Pre-Stress

Cues

The earliest recognition of a future stress problem
Worry and anticipation about future stress
Negative emotions such as anger, depression, and anxiety
Physical stress symptoms
Problem behaviors, reduced efficiency, and increased rigidity
Increased defensive, aggressive, or nonassertive behavior
A desire to avoid the situation

Goals

To anticipate what can be anticipated
To think through what I will have to think, do, and say
To focus on the specific task at hand
To combat self-defeating, irrational thinking
To emphasize planning and preparation
To relax when tension builds
To change what can be changed, and forget about that which cannot be changed

Mid-Stress

Cues

Recognition that the stress situation is at hand and that now is the best time to do something about it
Worry and anticipation about the situation
Negative emotions such as anger, depression, and anxiety
Physical stress symptoms
Problem behaviors, reduced efficiency, and increased rigidity
Increased defensive, aggressive, or nonassertive behavior

[1]Adapted by permission from Meichenbaum, D. (1985), *Stress inoculation training*. New York: Pergamon Press, pp. 72–73.

Goals

To solve problems and deal with the stress situation

To express what is on my mind

To reassure myself that I can handle the situation

To reinterpret stress as a constructive challenge, something to help me grow

To remain focused on the task

Post-Stress **Cues**

Recognition that the stress situation is essentially over
Worry and concern about what has happened
Negative emotions such as anger, depression, and anxiety
Physical stress symptoms
Problem behaviors, reduced efficiency, and increased rigidity
Increased defensive, aggressive, or nonassertive behavior

Goals

To evaluate my problem-solving strategies and identify what worked and what didn't

To find out what I can learn from this experience

To recognize that even small successes are important; to resist putting myself down for gradual progress

To praise myself for making an attempt to cope

To keep trying; not to expect complete success at once

To avoid "putting myself down" for setbacks and failures

To relax

Once you have identified your cues and coping goals for each phase, you are in a position to think of come-back strategies for coping with relapse. Here are a few general thoughts and actions others have suggested:

Pre-Stress Even if I can't anticipate what might happen, practicing getting into a problem-solving frame of mind is a good idea.
Now's the time to do my relaxation exercise. Now take a deep breath and relax.
It's normal to get tense before a stress situation.
Let's see if I can use this stress energy productively.
I'll set aside just 30 minutes for worrying and planning ahead.
All I can do is change what can be changed, and forget about the rest.
Just keep busy, it's better than wasting time getting upset.

Mid-Stress OK, it isn't the end of the world if I make a mistake.
I can use this as an opportunity to practice dealing with stress.
Just remember to use reason to deal with my fear.
One step at a time—I can deal with this.
Let's not get too personally involved.
Let's again take a constructive, problem-solving attitude.
Just sit back and think of all the alternative courses of action, then I'll make my choice.

There's no need to make more out of this than is necessary.
Don't focus on fear or anxiety, just what I have to do.
This anxiety (or anger) is normal.
Take care not to leap to conclusions.
Try not to blow things out of proportion.
Look for the positive; don't think negatively.
Relax. I'll use my relaxation exercises.

Post-Stress Even small successes are important.
It doesn't make sense to put myself down for gradual progress.
In learning new skills, it's normal to have ups and downs.
I may be upset, but I deserve a pat on the back for making an attempt to cope.
Sure, it felt bad. But it wasn't as bad as it could be.
This is not an absolute disaster; I'm making more out of the situation than it's worth.
So, it didn't work perfectly. I can accept that.
Next time I'll know what to expect, and can cope even better.
It doesn't make any sense to waste time putting myself down when things are over.

Fall-Back Strategies

To be perfectly honest, sometimes even come-back strategies do not work. It can be helpful to have thought through a final, fall-back strategy. We can see this in a particularly popular circus stunt (Smith, 1991):

> Imagine a tightrope walker at a circus. Although her performance might seem quite dangerous, she has a number of safety strategies. In case she slips, the balancing rod she carries can be used to latch onto the rope. She wears gloves that permit a stronger grip on the rope. If all these backups fail, there is a safety net to counter her fall. Similarly, in dealing with stress, think of a safety net strategy, what you can think and do if your backup coping strategies do not work.[2]

Fall-back strategies give you a useful safety net. For example, you might decide to talk to a friend, call a trusted relative, discuss the problem with a counselor, or write about what happened. Here are some additional fall-back thoughts:

Well, life goes on.
Everyone makes mistakes.
I still love myself (or have a loving family) in spite of my problems.
God still loves me.
Lets look at things in perspective.
Life is too short to make too much of this problem.
Maybe I'll learn from this somehow.

[2]Smith, J.C. (1991). *Stress Scripting*. New York: Praeger. p. 104.

Fall-back strategies help us go on living in the face of setbacks. They remind us not to put ourselves down for mistakes in thinking and behaving. And they prompt us to do better next time.

One fall-back strategy can be particularly useful when dealing with other people, especially when another person continues to behave aggressively (Chapter 18) or appears not to hear or understand what you want to say. Here, you might want to *process* what they are doing and ask why the other person isn't listening.

> Situation: Marcie's father has been pressuring her to go to graduate school. Marcie wants to take two years off to travel. She has explained this several times to her father, but he seems not to listen. He simply ignores what she is saying, and urges her to "stay on in school. I know what's best for you." Finally, when he did this for the ninth time, Marcie interrupted: "Father, for nine times you have ignored my wishes and simply ordered me to go on with school. I appreciate your concern for me, but it has become clear to me that we are not engaging in a discussion. Instead, you are just lecturing me. This frustrates me. I would much rather talk things through with you as two adults.

Fall-back Strategy

Cue: Complete failure of Marcie's assertion to be heard
Goal: To challenge her father on his failure to listen to her point of view
Fall-back Statement: "Father, for nine times you have ignored my wishes and simply ordered me to go on to school . . ."

Another fall-back strategy can be useful when the other person's defensive behavior is so upsetting to you that you cannot continue. Rather than abandon your script, announce that you are taking a break:

> Situation: James and Maurice have been lovers for five years. However, Maurice's mother objects. She complains that it is "against the Bible" for two men to love each other. One day she was having a heated discussion with James, who was getting so angry that he could barely think. But he knew he wanted to deal with the problem eventually. He decided to take time off, and announced, "I think we've talked enough about this for now. It is clear we haven't solved anything. However, I need a break."

Fall-back Strategy
Cue: James's anger and inability to think
Goal: To temporarily end the discussion, making it clear that there is still a disagreement.
Fall-back Statement: "I think we've talked enough . . ."

A more drastic fall-back strategy is to simply assert your point one final time, and close the discussion. This is illustrated below:

> Situation: Myrtle is frequently bothered by Chet's requests to borrow her car. She let him have it once, but regretted it because he returned it a day late. She has decided that from now on she will not lend her car to anyone. Chet persists in asking for the car. Myrtle carefully explains again and again why she would rather not let him have the car. When

he does not stop, she uses her fall-back strategy and simply announces, "We have talked about this long enough. You may not borrow my car, and that's that. Let's talk about something else."

Fall-back Strategy

Cue: Chet's persistence in asking to borrow the car
Goal: To stop discussion, and make one clear, final statement of why Myrtle will not lend the car
Fall-back Statement: "We have talked about this long enough . . ."

Stress Inoculation

Planning for possible relapse can actually contribute to the development of more powerful coping skills. The process is called *stress inoculation* (Meichenbaum, 1985). In medicine, we become inoculated against serious illness, say the flu or mumps, by receiving a small dose of the infectious agent. The body then develops a resistance that enables it to cope with exposure to the actual illness later on. Similarly, learning to cope with stress and relapse in a single stress situation can develop more general coping skills which can be applied to other situations. We become *inoculated* against stress. If you are interested in learning more about stress inoculation training, turn to Chapter 27.

Practice your come-back and fall-back strategies just as you would any coping strategy. You can use fantasy, role-play, or even diary notes (Chapters 3 through 5).

EXERCISE 25.1 *Identifying Potential Relapse*

Select a situation in which you are trying to cope better. What might go wrong? What type of relapse might occur?

What is a useful cue for this relapse?

What negative thinking might this cue trigger?

What coping thoughts would be more realistic and useful?

What are your come-back and fall-back strategies for this situation?

26

DESENSITIZING AND INOCULATING YOURSELF FOR STRESS

Target Coping Skills

- Combining stress management skills to reduce stress in specific situations

Purpose

- Fears and phobias
- Anxiety in interpersonal situations
- Performance and test anxiety

Example

Violet has an intense fear of public speaking. She avoids talking in front of groups whenever possible. Applying stress inoculation training, she conditioned herself to experience public speaking with less anxiety. This involved first developing a list of ten public speaking situations, ranked from least to most stressful. Then, for each situation, she practiced imagining the initial danger cue of walking up to a podium and thinking the negative, anxiety-arousing thoughts that followed. In each practice session, she would then relax deeply so that the anxiety would go away. She then proceeded to rehearse thoughts that were more rational and useful and ended with a reward. CUE → COPE → REWARD Summary: PODIUM + NEGATIVE THINKING → RELAXATION + COPING THOUGHTS → REWARD

Many forms of stress management involve directly confronting a stress situation. For example, to be assertive, you state your thoughts and feelings to another person. To manage time, you face your priorities and obligations. However, what happens when stress situations are so anxiety-arousing that it is difficult to face them in the first place? Such situations often call for desensitization and stress inoculation training, two popular approaches to stress management that combine many already covered in this book.

Some of the ideas central to desensitization and stress inoculation training are just common sense advice. Take, for example, the following:

Focus on one problem at a time.

Deal with things when you are calm and in a good mood.

Do not try to solve everything at once.

Do not bite off more than you can chew.

If things get too bad, just take a break to recover.

Desensitization and stress inoculation training can be seen as systematic and scientifically based applications of such notions. In addition, they integrate many of the stress management strategies we have already considered, especially problem solving, assertiveness training, cognitive restructuring, and relaxation training. For desensitization and stress inoculation training to work, you need to have covered Chapters 1 through 5, as well as the following:

Cognitive Stress

Chapter 6: Catching Stressful Thoughts

Chapter 7: Changing Stressful Assumptions and Beliefs

Chapter 8: Reducing Worry

Relaxation

Chapter 11: Practicing Physical Relaxation Techniques

Chapter 12: Practicing Mental Relaxation

Chapter 14: Making a Relaxation Script or Tape

Interpersonal Skill Problems

Chapter 15: Developing Relationships

Chapter 16: Making Requests, Saying No, and Dealing with Conflicts

Chapter 17: Dealing with Your Anger

Chapter 18: Dealing with Aggression

Relapse Prevention

Chapter 25: Preventing Relapse

Desensitization

Desensitization was formally introduced by Joseph Wolpe in 1958. Initially, it was designed as a treatment for *phobias*—serious and often incapacitating fears that have no basis in reality. Common phobias include the fear of crowds, heights, open places, strangers, tests, and doctors. It should be noted that a true phobia is truly irrational, that is, the feared object is not really dangerous and the phobic person may have the skills to cope, but is too anxious to use them.

The desensitization procedure is fairly simple. First, you master an approach to relaxation. Then you identify a stressful situation you find difficult to handle. Be concrete and specific, identifying the critical moments.

Next, generate ten versions of this situation and rank them from least to most stressful. This is your desensitization hierarchy. For example, a hierarchy of 10 stimuli relating to a fear of heights might include:

1. Watching someone else climb a ladder (least fear-arousing)
2. Standing on a firm chair
3. Starting to climb a ladder
4. Climbing halfway up a ladder
5. Standing on top of a ladder
6. Taking an elevator to the top of a tall building
7. Standing on top of a one-story building
8. Standing on top of a tall building inside a glass-enclosed room
9. Standing in the middle of the roof of a tall building, several feet from the railing
10. Standing on the roof of a tall building looking out over the railing (most fear-arousing)

Students often have trouble selecting ten versions of one target situation and, instead, confuse a number of target situations. For example one coping team member, Judy, included the following situations among her ten:

7. Paying for an item, then immediately discovering a defect and asking for an exchange
8. Calling up a store to complain about a defective purchase
9. Taking an item back to the store for a refund
10. Asking my boss for a raise

Although Judy thought that "asking my boss for a raise" fit into this hierarchy because it was a stressful example of making requests, the item does not really belong. Can you see why? Obviously, each of the other items has to do with assertively making an adjustment concerning a defective purchase. When you select a concrete and specific stress situation, the other examples on your hierarchy *should involve the same situation*. Judy would need to develop a different hierarchy for "asking my boss for a raise." Sample items might include:

7. Asking my boss for a different lamp
8. Asking my boss for a different desk
9. Asking my boss for a room change
10. Asking my boss for a raise

Once you have your hierarchy, you can begin desensitization. First you relax. Make sure you are really relaxed. Then start imagining the least anxiety-arousing situation on the hierarchy (looking at someone else climb a ladder). Include every detail, in proper sequence. Where are you? Who is there? What are you doing? What are you thinking? What happens next?

You continue imagining this situation until you feel the first signs of anxiety. At this point, you stop imagining your situation and start relaxing again until you are completely calm. Then begin again with the same situation. When you can imagine the complete situation two or three times without becoming anxious, you can graduate to the next fearful situation (standing on a firm chair) and repeat the imagination-relaxation process. Never cover more than two situations in any one session. Eventually every situation on the hierarchy will be covered.

Desensitization appears to work by means of two processes. First, feelings of fear are replaced by feelings of relaxation. Why? Because relaxation is consistently paired with fear, stimuli that evoke fear eventually evoke its opposite, relaxation. This is called *counterconditioning*. Second, by gently confronting a fearful stimulus, the client learns that it is not as dangerous as originally seemed. Fear weakens or *extinguishes*.

Stress Inoculation Training

Stress inoculation training (Meichenbaum, 1985), as we noted in a previous chapter, is something like a vaccination. For example, an influenza vaccination consists of a small and harmless dose of the flu virus. The body responds to this dose by building up a resistance sufficiently strong to combat actual exposure to the flu. Similarly, in stress inoculation training, you are exposed to a relatively innocuous version of a stressful situation. You respond by building up coping skills that then can be applied to more severe stressors later on.

Like desensitization, stress inoculation training incorporates relaxation and graduated exposure. However, it can also incorporate many of the stress management strategies we have already considered. This occurs in three phases:

Conceptualization Phase. In the first phase, you conceptualize your problem in terms of stress management. This involves reading Chapters 1 through 5.

Skill Phase. There are many skills you may apply in stress inoculation training. These include relaxation, catching and replacing irrational and self-defeating thoughts, assertiveness, and relapse prevention.

Application and Follow-Through Phase. This phase is most like desensitization. Here, you rehearse applying the skills you acquired. You might practice being assertive in certain situations, relaxing, or replacing negative statements to yourself with coping statements. As in desensitization, you construct a *hierarchy* of increasingly stressful situations and then rehearse each while relaxed. However, in stress inoculation training, make sure that two to four of your situations are *relapse situations* (Chapter 24). For example, our hierarchy regarding fear of heights has been revised to include three relapse situations:

1. Watching someone else climb a ladder (least fear-arousing)
2. **Relapse situation:** Standing on a firm chair; thinking, "This isn't going to help me. I don't know what I'm doing. I still feel anxious."; climbing down from the chair
3. Starting to climb a ladder
4. **Relapse situation:** Climbing halfway up a ladder; thinking, "I can feel my stomach getting tense. This means I'm going to panic. I haven't learned a thing. I'll fail. I have to stop."
5. Standing on top of a ladder
6. Taking an elevator to the top of a tall building
7. Standing on top of a one-story building
8. Standing on top of a tall building inside a glass-enclosed room
9. **Relapse situation:** Standing in the middle of the roof of a tall building, several feet from the railing; getting anxious, thinking "I'm sure I'm going to fall. I can't take this," and climbing down the stairs
10. Standing on the roof of a tall building looking out over the railing (most fear-arousing)

In stress inoculation, what you do with each situation is a little different from desensitization. Mental rehearsal involves thinking through what you will think and do in each of the situations in your hierarchy. It is a special type of fantasy that involves five stages:

- Note cues: You imagine cues that indicate that stress is beginning to build. These are signals to start coping.
- Note self-defeating, irrational thoughts: Actually start thinking the negative, stress-producing thoughts that you have identified as part of your problem.
- Stop and relax: Negative thoughts are stopped (perhaps through the thought stopping techniques in Chapter 8), and then you relax.
- Think coping thoughts and behaviors: Now, think some statements to yourself that are useful and rational. Apply some coping skills.
- Evaluate and review yourself: Think back over the stressful encounter, and reward yourself for skills that have been applied and identify what specific skills might be applied better.

This sequence should be a bit familiar to you. It is essentially an elaboration of the 1 → 2 → 3 COPE system we described in Chapter 4. Recall the steps:

CUE

↓

COPE

↓

REWARD

We have expanded the cope stage to include:

CUE

↓

Note Self-Defeating Irrational Behavior

Stop and relax.

Think Coping Thoughts and Behaviors

↓

REWARD

This may seem a bit complicated, but such application is actually something of a coping fantasy, one you may already have entertained. Here is how one person might visualize dealing with the stress of taking an exam.

Cue	I can visualize the instructor passing out the exams. He has just given the instructions. I have my pencil in hand and am holding my breath. He hands me an exam, and my heart begins to
Irrational, Self-Defeating Thoughts	beat wildly. I start thinking, "This exam is so long, I'll never finish! Look! Everyone else seems so calm! I can't go through with this." Wait! Handing me an exam—that's my cue to use the coping skills I rehearsed ear-
Stop and Relax	lier. I imagine myself thinking, "Hey, just a minute. Close your eyes and slowly squeeze your shoulders and let
Coping Thoughts and Behaviors	go. Relax. Just answer one question at a time. Skip those you can't answer, and return to them later. One at a time and skip the hard ones—
Reward & Evaluation	that's my coping rule." Good. I remembered my relaxation exercise and coping thought. Now to begin.

The rehearsal of coping skills does not always have to be just imagined. The client and counselor can act out stressful scenarios in role-playing. Or, both may agree on homework assignments in which preselected real-life stressors are confronted. Once again, it is important to attempt such practice with the assistance of a trained mental health professional.

EXERCISE 26.1 *Stress Inoculation*

1. Identify a concrete, specific, and realistic stress situation.
2. Think of ten versions of this situation, including from two to four relapse situations.
3. Rank these from least (1) to most (10) stressful.
4. Generally, what will you include in each step of your mental rehearsal?

- Note cues: You imagine cues that indicate that stress is beginning to build. These are signals to start coping.
- Note self-defeating, irrational thoughts: Actually start thinking the negative, stress-producing thoughts that you have identified as part of your problem.
- Stop and Relax: Negative thoughts are stopped (perhaps through the thought-stopping techniques in Chapter 8), and then you relax.
- Think coping thoughts and behaviors: Now, think some statements to yourself that are useful and rational. Apply some coping skills.
- Evaluate and Reward Yourself: Think back over the stressful encounter, and reward yourself for skills that have been applied and identify what specific skills might be applied better.

5. Now, engage in your fantasy. Start imagining your first stressful situation. On a scale from 1 to 10, where 1 means "not at all stressed," 10 means "maximum stress," and five means "intermediate level of stress," what number would you give yourself?
6. Continue with your fantasy, incorporating the 5 steps just considered.
7. When finished with your fantasy, rate your stress level again on a ten-point scale.
8. Repeat from three to five times, until your stress level has gone down by at least two points.

27

DEFENDING YOURSELF WHEN SITUATIONS CANNOT BE CHANGED

Target Coping Skills

- Distinguishing between appropriate and inappropriate defensive strategies
- Learning what to do when everything else fails

Purpose

- Reduction of pain and discomfort of unavoidable stress
- Gaining "buying time" to figure out how to cope

Example

Reggi has just been diagnosed as having AIDS (Acquired Immune Deficiency Syndrome). He is overwhelmed with all sorts of feelings and is not sure what to do. Some days he stays home and sits in the corner. Eventually, when he finds himself sitting alone, he decides to let himself think, "Things may be OK. I'm sure they're working on a cure." Somewhat reassured, he feels less confused and helpless. He resumes work and seeks medical help. CUE → COPE → REWARD Summary: SITTING ALONE → THOUGHTS THAT "THINGS MAY BE OK" → FEELINGS OF BEING REASSURED AND LESS HELPLESS

Here is a challenging idea: Sometimes it is better *not* to attempt to cope with stress. You might think this contradicts everything this book has been saying. But some situations call for cost-containment strategies. Consider these examples:

> Brenda has just broken up with her boyfriend. The painful facts are that she will now have to pay for her own rent, look for a job and live alone.

> Tomorrow she has an important job interview. Rather than cope with the complexities of her serious situation, she thinks, "Things are OK. My boyfriend will come back. I don't have to make plans for living alone." Brenda's temporary denial of the facts enables her to focus all her attention on her interview and do her best.
>
> Jody has just undergone surgery for breast cancer. There are many things that could concern her, such as the possibility of recurrence, the loss of time from work to recover, and the disfiguring effects of surgery. However, for a month Jody lives in a state of calm indifference. By not facing the facts, she is able to enjoy a certain degree of peace, one that may well minimize the destructive effects of stress on the healing process.

Neither Brenda nor Jody actively coped with their problems. Indeed, both could be said to be avoiding some very unpleasant facts. However, sometimes such avoidance is an important defensive strategy. Defense can provide us with a breathing spell to collect our resources for future coping efforts. It can enable us to relax and recover from potentially destructive levels of tension. It can provide a "positive illusion" of being in control when things may well be out of our control (Taylor, 1989). Finally, some stress situations simply cannot be changed and the best we can do is protect ourselves and go on living.

The importance of strategic defense is particularly evident in many crises. Marti Horowitz (1976) has described the stages through which victims of tragedy pass. First, one experiences an outcry of anguish or a period of denial. In denial the problem is simply put out of mind. The individual might even feel "numb" or disinterested in life as a way of avoiding thinking about a crisis. Next comes a period of intrusiveness in which there is a flood of thoughts and pangs of anguish about the crisis. This can include nightmares as well as obsessive preoccupation.

Horowitz emphasizes that repeated cycles of denial and intrusiveness can actually help to work through a crisis. In each intrusive phase, the individual is "dosed" with a small aspect of a tragedy to think about. This is followed by a period of denial which serves as something of a rest period to prevent becoming overwhelmed with pain and despair. Denial is then followed by another period of intrusiveness so that more of the problem can be dealt with. Eventually, through manageable doses, one learns to accept the crisis event as reality and then go on living. We can see that defensive denial can be an absolutely essential part of coping with severe stress.

Suzanne Miller (1987) has proposed a related way of looking at defense. She has suggested that people differ in their preferred ways of dealing with information about stress. For example, if you are about to undergo dental surgery, should the dentist explain the details of the procedure and its possible effects, or should you be encouraged to divert your attention and think about something completely unrelated? According to Miller, the answer depends on whether you are a *monitor* or a *blunter*. Monitors prefer to seek information about a threat, whereas blunters prefer to seek distraction from a threat. A monitor would prefer to be well informed about an upcoming dental procedure, whereas a blunter would prefer not to know (and indeed have attention diverted from the procedure). Research on the significance of these two styles is still underway and may help us determine if monitors generally do better than blunters, or if it is better to pick the strategy one prefers.

Healthy and Unhealthy Defense

The goals of defense are self-protection and containment of the potential damage of stress. When no other options are available, defense can be a useful response. However, defensive strategies can be a problem when they are automatic habits outside of our control, or when they distort perception and interfere with coping options that may be available.

Norma Haan (1965, 1977) has suggested a useful way of viewing some of the more widely used defense strategies. Each can be an excessive or distorted application of a coping strategy. For example, the coping strategy *concentration* enables us to focus on a task at hand and ignore potentially disruptive feelings of anxiety. During a job interview you may choose to focus your attention on each question asked by the interviewer rather than on your own performance. The same process of concentration can be a potentially destructive defense strategy if you simply refuse to face or accept an unpleasant reality. Here, concentration is *denial.* Denial is self-destructive when you avoid taking actions necessary for your well-being, such as denying that a serious cough might be pneumonia requiring a visit to the doctor. Additional defense and coping strategies are outlined in Table 27-1.

There is a time and place for defense mechanisms. This can be clearly seen in the case of denial. First of all, denial involves refusing to admit that something exists. You can deny that you are hurt, that things are going badly, that you need to start planning or that nothing is working out. Lazarus has suggested some rules for when it is OK to deny (Lazarus & Folkman, 1984):

- When you simply can't do anything about a problem, you might as well ignore it in order to feel better ("I am terminally ill, and that cannot be changed.")
- Sometimes denying certain parts of a problem can help you cope better with others. ("My heart disease is a threat to my life. Rather than dwelling on that, I will pay very diligent attention to keeping up with my medications and diet.")
- When a problem will never happen again, minimize the costs of not coping. ("I really don't want to spend time helping this volunteer organization. But, I doubt they will ever ask me again, so, I'll just deny to myself that it's a problem.)
- Denial may well be helpful at an early stage of a long and complicated problem, especially if you have limited energy, time, and other resources to cope with every stage. Such denial may well give you some needed time off or breathing room to develop better coping resources.

TABLE 27-1 Defense and Coping Mechanisms

COPING PROCESS: Objectivity (realistically and rationally separating thoughts and feelings). EXAMPLE: John is upset over having lost a job. Rather than let his feelings interfere with looking for a new job, he thinks, "Sometimes I feel like a failure. However, tonight I will put my feelings aside and plan how to find a new job."	DEFENSE PROCESS: Isolation (unconsciously separating thoughts and feelings that belong together so their connection is not seen). EXAMPLE: John hides from his feelings of being upset. He thinks, "Well, what happens, happens," and appears on the surface to be unconcerned.
COPING PROCESS: Logical analysis (careful thinking through of problems and their causes). EXAMPLE: Sally has lost her keys. She thinks, "Now let's figure this out. Let's retrace my steps today."	DEFENSE PROCESS: Rationalization (creating a logical-sounding explanation in order to hide painful feelings) EXAMPLE: Sally thinks, "My keys aren't really lost. I just put them somewhere hard to find so they wouldn't be stolen."

TABLE 27-1 (*Continued*)

COPING PROCESS: Tolerance of ambiguity (continuing to cope even when things are unsure). EXAMPLE: Nate has to write a term paper and is not sure which topic is best. He starts to work anyway because he knows that his ideas will get clearer as he continues to work.	DEFENSE PROCESS: Severe doubt and indecision (feeling psychologically paralyzed so that you simply cannot act or make up your mind just because all the information is not in). EXAMPLE: Nate spends hours considering various term paper topics even though he gets nowhere.
COPING PROCESS: Concentration (setting aside disturbing thoughts and feelings in order to effectively complete what you are doing). EXAMPLE: Joan has just moved away from home. She is homesick and lonely, but puts these feelings aside so she can study and pass her courses.	DEFENSE PROCESS: Denial (refusing to recognize events, thoughts, and feelings that are upsetting). EXAMPLE: Joan thinks to herself, "No, I haven't really moved away from home. This is just a temporary vacation. And I'm not really upset."
COPING PROCESS: Empathy (accurately sensing and telling others you understand what they are thinking and feeling). EXAMPLE: Maurice is talking to a very irate customer. He comments, "I can tell you are very upset because the item you want isn't in."	DEFENSE PROCESS: Projection (denying the existence of your own thoughts, feelings or motives, while wrongly ascribing these thoughts to other people). EXAMPLE: Maurice, who doesn't realize he is angry at his co-worker for leaving early last week, listens to his co-worker's general complaints. George inaccurately thinks, "Why is he so angry at me?"
COPING PROCESS: Regression in the service of the ego (exhibiting creative, childlike playfulness in a healthy manner). EXAMPLE: Sonja and Bruce are trying to plan a trip this summer. They can think of where to go. Suddenly, they start playing around and have fun thinking of silly ideas. "Let's go to Mars, or to the bottom of the ocean."	DEFENSE PROCESS: Regression (retreating to earlier and less mature patterns of behavior in order to avoid present threat). EXAMPLE: After Bruce disagrees with her suggestions, Sonja goes to a corner and starts pouting like a child.
COPING PROCESS: Sublimation (finding a satisfying and appropriate substitution for urges that may be threatening or inappropriate if directly expressed). EXAMPLE: Edward is sexually excited by his teacher. He knows how inappropriate it would be to approach her. He finds a substitute by reading romance stories.	DEFENSE PROCESS: Displacement (less satisfying and maladaptive substitutions are found for pent-up feelings). EXAMPLE: Edward, excited by his teacher, begins compulsively dating older, married women.
COPING PROCESS: Substitution (deliberately doing one thing instead of what you want to do, because of the demands of the situation). EXAMPLE: Grace has just been hired as a clerk. The first week her supervisor asks her to go out and buy flowers for his wife. She feels like screaming at him but wants to keep the job. She decides to get the flowers, a deliberate compromise.	DEFENSE PROCESS: Reaction formation (blocking awareness of one threatening feeling by unconsciously doing the opposite). EXAMPLE: Grace hides her anger from herself and her boss by smiling and saying, "I want to help in every way I can. I really enjoy these little extra jobs you have for me."
COPING PROCESS: Suppression (deliberately putting aside thoughts and feelings that may be unsuitable or uncomfortable). EXAMPLE: Hector is interviewing for a job. His prospective boss is wearing a very ugly and amusing tie. Hector suppresses the urge to laugh, and simply goes on with the interview.	DEFENSE PROCESS: Repression (unconsciously blocking painful thoughts and feelings). EXAMPLE: Hector does not get the job. Deep down inside he is hurt. However, he does not want to admit this to himself and goes on as if it did not matter to him.

- It may be less dangerous to deny things that are very ambiguous in the first place. ("I'm only ten pounds over my ideal weight. I don't have a weight problem).

Researchers (Carver, Scheier, & Weintraum, 1989; Lazarus & Folman, 1984) have suggested some other strategies that, like denial, may be helpful or harmful. Some involve accepting reality, but changing how we view it. These include:

Accepting reality: which involves accepting and living with the fact that a stressful event has occurred, is real, and cannot be changed.

Accepting responsibility: which involves assuming that one has brought the problem on oneself.

Positive reinterpretation and growth: involves reappraising a stressful situation in positive terms, that is, looking for the "silver lining" of a stressful situation and seeing how it might contribute to learning and growth.

Other strategies involve some form of substitute satisfaction or tension release:

Seeking social support for emotional reasons: is seeking moral support, sympathy, or understanding.

Seeking alternative rewards: involves changing one's activities in order to obtain satisfactions not available in a stressful encounter.

Turning to religion: by praying as well as seeking and trusting in "God's help."

Focusing on and venting emotions: involves focusing on one's feelings of being upset and expressing them.

Reducing tension: involves disengaging from a stressful situation through relaxation, jogging, or exercise.

Resorting to humor: involves laughing at, joking about, and making fun of a stressful situation.

Still other forms involve some distortion or withdrawal from the facts of a stressful situation.

Wishful thinking: involves simply wishing or hoping a stressful situation will change or go away.

Behavioral disengagement: involves giving up attempts to attain the goal because of the stressor's interference.

Mental disengagement: involves becoming psychologically disengaged from the goal through substitute activities like watching TV, daydreaming, sleeping, or becoming distracted.

Self-isolation: involves avoiding people in general and keeping others from knowing how bad things are.

Alcohol/drug use: involves disengaging from a stressor by using alcohol or other drugs.

Some of these are obviously more dangerous than others. And some could well contribute to potentially effective coping. Can you tell the difference?

EXERCISE 26.1 ***Costs and Benefits of Defense***

Take a look at the defensive strategies listed in this chapter. Which have you used? What have been their costs and benefits to you?

28

COPING WITH PAIN

Target Coping Skills

- Managing pain

Purpose

- Acute (intense, short-term) pain
- Chronic (long-lasting) pain

Example

Ken suffers from a chronic backache. Often it prevents him from devoting full attention to his work and to his family. In attempting to deal with his pain, Ken first kept a daily diary of his pain episodes and what happened immediately before. He discovered two patterns: his backaches got worse after three hours of sitting at work, and whenever his wife would ask him to do additional work at home. Sitting at work was an easy warning sign to manage. He decided that after sitting down at work for 45 minutes, he would then stand up and walk around. Also, whenever his wife would ask him to do additional work at home, he would not passively agree. Instead, he would assertively suggest that they negotiate a reasonable division of work. Ken decided to permit himself the pleasure of a good cup of coffee each time he remembered to put his coping plans into action. CUE → COPE → REWARD Summaries: PERIOD OF SITTING DOWN → WALK AROUND OFFICE → COFFEE; REQUEST TO WORK AT HOME → SUGGESTION TO NEGOTIATE → COFFEE

Here is one stress experience which nearly everyone has had—pain. Whether it be a toothache, headache, backache, injury, or burn, pain is a truly universal experience. We will consider two types of pain: acute and chronic.

Acute pain, by definition, lasts a short time and may be helped with a mild pain-killing medication. It typically has a clear cause, such as a burn, injury or physical disorder. In contrast, chronic pain lasts much longer, usually at least six months, and often has an obscure cause. Examples include chronic headaches, backaches and joint pain. People who suffer chronic pain have often tried to get medical or surgical help, without relief. They may become dependent on addicting pain-killers, and may even develop a variety of self-defeating coping strategies (drinking, avoiding work, social isolation) in an attempt to ease their afflictions.

Chronic pain can be a considerable frustration because there is often no underlying pathology, or if there is, the pathology itself is chronic. If no medical cause for your pain can be found, you may have been told that the pain is "all in the head," that it is somehow less than real. Yet most pain victims feel their pain is quite real indeed.

Perhaps a more useful approach is to accept that all pain is real, and is the result of many complicated factors. A number of examples make this point very clear. First, the severity of pain depends on how it is interpreted. In World War II, a young medical corp physician, Howard Beecher (1959) noted that only about a quarter of seriously injured men requested pain killers. In contrast, about 80 percent of civilian patients with similar wounds requested painkillers. A possible explanation is that, for patients and soldiers, pain has different meanings: a soldier may see pain as a sign that he is alive and may be sent home; for a civilian pain can mean that unpleasant treatment may be required and life will be interrupted. The negative or positive meanings attributed to pain help determine its intensity.

The way in which we direct our attention can also influence the experience of pain. A hospitalized patient, alone and preoccupied with pain, may experience considerable discomfort. In contrast, a movie actor, concentrating on his or her lines, may be totally unaware of an injured foot.

One theory helps make sense out of such unusual experiences. Melzack and Wall (1965, 1982) describe a neurological "gate" in the spinal cord that modulates the flow of nerve signals from the body to the brain. The experience of pain depends on whether or not this gate is closed or open. Surprisingly, a variety of factors can "close" the gate and lessen pain, including:

- Good skills for coping with other stressors
- Active involvement in tasks
- Concentration on stimuli other than oneself and one's pain
- Reduced physical tension
- Positive emotional states
- Pain-coping strategies that help one feel "in control"

Factors that can "open" the gate of pain include:

- Poor coping skills in general
- Self-involvement and preoccupation with one's pain
- Passive withdrawal
- Increased physical tension
- Negative emotional states such as depression, anger, and anxiety
- Lack of effective pain-coping strategies

In this chapter we will consider the wide range of strategies people use to "close" the gate of pain (Hanson & Gerber, 1990). It is helpful to note that the more strategies you have available and have practiced, the better you will be able to manage pain. Before beginning any pain management program, it is absolutely essential that you consult a physician to assess any physical problem that may be causing your pain and if the coping strategies you are considering may affect your physical condition.

Develop Good General Coping Skills

All of the coping strategies considered in this book could be part of a pain-management program. The reason is that poor coping skills lead to increased stress which, in turn, can aggravate pain. Simple stress arousal can direct our attention to pain, amplify the pain we experience, and even aggravate physical conditions that are the source of pain (for example, a burn patient may nervously scratch his or her skin under stress, aggravating a painful wound; a backache patient may slump over in his or her chair under stress, aggravating a back condition.)

Relaxation exercises (Chapters 10 through 14) can be particularly useful for dealing with pain. Such exercises can divert attention, reduce arousal, and provide an increased sense of control over pain. Of these, isometric squeeze relaxation (Chapter 11) may be of less use than other exercises. However, developing a relaxation script (Chapter 14) for pain may be especially helpful.

Identify Pain Triggers

It can be useful to consider pain as a stress symptom, and look for critical moments and early warning signs as cues or "pain triggers." Such triggers can include certain physical activities that tax physical as well as psychological capacities. For certain types of headache, early warning signs can also include "prodromal" symptoms such as increased sensitivity to light. Often people respond to pain triggers in ways that aggravate, or at best fail to significantly reduce, pain. These include thinking catastrophically ("I can't stand the pain"), engaging in imagery that increases the vividness of the pain experience ("It feels like my hand is burning up"), or withdrawing from people or activities. Once a pain trigger is identified, consider an appropriate coping response and reward using the CUE → COPE → REWARD system. Here are some coping strategies many have found useful:

- Redefine the pain
- Transform the pain in fantasy
- Divert your attention
- Attend to the pain
- Express your feelings about the pain

Redefine the Pain

Often our thoughts and beliefs can aggravate pain by directing our attention to it and ascribing negative meaning to it. For this reason, one step in pain management is to counter such thinking as:

"This pain is the end of the world."

"I simply can't stand this."

"There is nothing I can do to escape; therefore I am doomed to live in misery."

"Things just seem completely hopeless."

"Pain and discomfort are always unhealthy. This is not good for me. I'm going to suffer the consequences."

Each of us defines pain in our own way. Pain might be a signal of underlying pathology (even though none may be present), an indicator of one's helplessness, or an excuse to avoid unpleasant tasks. Often, our definitions actually aggravate and prolong pain. If we are convinced of some undiagnosed pathology or of our helplessness, pain may seem serious indeed. And if pain is rewarded with "secondary" gains, it is likely to persist.

Hanson and Gerber (1990) offer three very useful ways of redefining pain. Pain can be viewed as a *teacher*, or a reminder, of the need to acquire more effective coping skills. When viewed as such, it is important not to think punitive or excessively self-critical thoughts. Examples of helpful self-statements include:

"What is my pain teaching me?"

"There's a lesson in my pain—I overdid it yesterday when playing sports."

"I must be getting too emotionally upset. That's why my pain is getting worse."

"I can now perfect my relaxation and coping skills."

Pain can also be viewed as an unusual *challenge to "go with the flow."* The more you resist pain, the more pain-aggravating tension you create. Yet giving up completely also creates feelings of helplessness and depression, which can also aggravate pain. Think of pain as a storm. A storm cannot be stopped or prevented, but it can be weathered. Similarly, you may not be able to stop pain, but you can weather it. Another image is that of a surfer floating on the waves. It would be disaster for the surfer to try to push away or fight waves, even those that seem to get in the way. Instead, the surfer learns to flow with and ride each wave. Learn to flow with pain. In accepting the challenge of pain, remember, like any big storm, pain is time-limited. It cannot last forever. Here are some examples of helpful statements:

"I can survive this because it will be over soon."

"I've experienced this pain before. I know I can live with it."

"Stay calm. Breathe slowly and deeply. Don't push the pain. Just calmly accept it and go on working."

Finally, pain can also be seen as "a very tricky *enemy* that must be fought skillfully." This enemy uses a variety of weapons, including: getting you upset and tense, making you feel helpless, interfering with life and enjoyment, making you feel isolated or turning you into a drug addict or alcoholic. The more successful the pain is at using these weapons, the more of a grip it has on you. You have to learn how to fight pain skillfully, using careful pain-management and stress management skills, such as saying:

"I'm not going to let this pain get the best of me."

"My pain is up to its old tricks again."

"I'll fight back the pain. I now know what to do."

"Go ahead and hurt me; I'll show you who's on top."

"I bet you want me to get into drugs. Well, I'm on to you. I know your tricks."

"You're trying to get me upset and make me forget what I'm doing. I'll just ignore you."

Transform the Pain through Fantasy

Mental imagery is a powerful tool (Chapter 12). Many people find it useful to use fantasy to transform the experience of pain. You might imagine you are in a situation in which your pain has a more positive meaning:

"I think that I am a soldier carrying out an important mission. My leg injury hurts, but doesn't stop me."

"I imagine myself as a sports star. The game is nearly over. I experience my pain, but I can handle it."

You might also fantasize an imaginary cause for your pain. Picture your pain caused by imaginary electricity, nerves being stretched or tied up in knots, vices clamping on the body, or burning flames. At first, you might wonder about the point of vividly imagining such causes. Once you picture an imaginary cause, then, in your fantasy, *modify* the cause to reduce the pain. Turn down the electricity, loosen the knots, release the vice and extinguish the flames. Remember, you are using the vast powers of the imagination to transform pain.

Finally, imagine a sensation that is roughly similar to your pain, but one you can tolerate better. If you think about it, pain sensations can be rather like sensations of heat, cold, and numbness. Imagine your pain as sensations of heat evoked by the intense sun, cold caused by ice on your skin, or numbness caused by the injection of a pain-killer.

Divert Your Attention

Pain gets our attention. This, of course, is highly desirable. The child learns quickly to remove his or her finger from the fire. Pain tells us to remove a potentially damaging condition or to seek help. We often hesitate to seek distraction from our pain because we have been taught to take pain seriously.

Yet distraction can be an effective strategy for coping with chronic pain. It is extremely difficult to attend to several stimuli at once. If you attend to stimuli other than pain, there is simply less attention left for pain. Hanson and Gerber (1990) describe a simple experiment you can do to demonstrate this:

> Just close your eyes and become very aware of some part of your body that you associate with pain. Notice carefully the sensations coming from that part right now. What do those sensations feel like? . . . (pause) . . . And now open your eyes and begin looking very closely at . . . (name some object in the room). Look at it closely, noticing its size, shape, and color. Try to focus all of your attention, all of your awareness right now on this object. . . . Just keep studying it as though you were seeing it for the first time . . .[1]

Particularly useful are highly active forms of distraction, including work, recreation (such as sports and hobbies), and social activities (Sternbach, 1987). Of course, you should maintain a balance between work and play (Chapter 9) and do not attempt activities that will aggravate your pain. Also, the more serious your pain, the more complex the distracting activity should be. Completing a simple crossword puzzle may work for a minor ache. But if the ache gets worse, you may have to find a more demanding and involving activity.

You can even divert your attention to relatively mundane or neutral mental activities, including:

- Planning your day's schedule
- Making a shopping list
- Memorizing a list of new words

[1]Hanson, R. W., and Gerber, K. E. (1990). *Coping with Chronic Pain*. New York: Guilford, p. 106.

It is also possible to direct your attention to everyday activities that you usually do in an automatic manner:

- Taking a shower
- Brushing your teeth
- Dressing and undressing
- Driving or walking to a familiar place

Hanson and Gerber suggest thinking of such a continuous deployment of attention as a way of "building concentration" or "developing meditative skills" (See Chapter 12). That is, meditatively maintain your attention on a diversion rather than pain.

Attend to the Pain This strategy may seem a bit paradoxical. How can attending to pain help us cope? However, the key is to simply attend to your pain in a way that is calm and dispassionate. You might attempt to figure out different aspects of your discomfort, as if you were a scientist or doctor. You might notice that this approach involves the defensive strategies of emotional insulation and intellectualization. However, by focusing on the pain you do demonstrate something about the nature of pain—it can often be tolerated.

Express Your Feelings about Pain Finally, it can be useful to talk to someone about your pain. Look for chances to talk about your feelings. Talk about your pain and discomfort with someone who is empathic. This person should ideally care about your feelings and show some understanding. You also might consider putting your feelings about pain into words or pictures. For example, you might write a letter, diary entry, poem, or song about your feelings. Another strategy would be to make a drawing or sketch.

EXERCISE 28.1 *Pain Log: Old Coping Strategies*

In the space below, describe the nature of your pain problem.

In the following log, identify when you experience pain, the intensity of the pain, and possible critical moments and early warning signs (what you were doing before that could possibly have contributed to the pain). In describing intensity, use this "0 to 5" scale:

0 = No pain whatsoever

1 = Mild pain, aware of it only when attending to it

2 = Mild pain, can be ignored at times

3 = Moderate pain, noticeably present

4 = Severe pain, makes it difficult to concentrate; can do undemanding tasks

5 = Extremely intense pain; cannot concentrate or do anything

Then, describe your old coping strategies, and indicate how effective they are.

	SUNDAY	MONDAY	TUESDAY	WEDNESDAY	THURSDAY	FRIDAY	SATURDAY
Possible critical moment							
Possible warning sign							
Intensity of pain before trying to cope							
Old coping strategy							
Outcome of coping strategy, including intensity of pain after trying to cope							

EXERCISE 28.2 *Pain Log: New Coping Strategies*

In this log, record various new coping strategies you have tried for coping with pain. Again, indicate when you experience pain, the intensity of the pain, and possible critical moments and early warning signs (what you were doing before that could possibly have contributed to the pain). In describing intensity, use this "0 to 5" scale:

0 = No pain whatsoever

1 = Mild pain, aware of it only when attending to it

2 = Mild pain, can be ignored at times

3 = Moderate pain, noticeably present

4 = Severe pain, makes it difficult to concentrate; can do undemanding tasks

5 = Extremely intense pain; cannot concentrate or do anything

Then, describe your coping strategies, and indicate how effective they are, and the rewards you have selected for coping.

	SUNDAY	MONDAY	TUESDAY	WEDNESDAY	THURSDAY	FRIDAY	SATURDAY
Possible critical moment							
Possible warning sign							
Intensity of pain before trying to cope							
Coping strategy							
Outcome of coping strategy, including intensity of pain. What worked? What could you improve upon?							
Reward selected for attempting to cope							

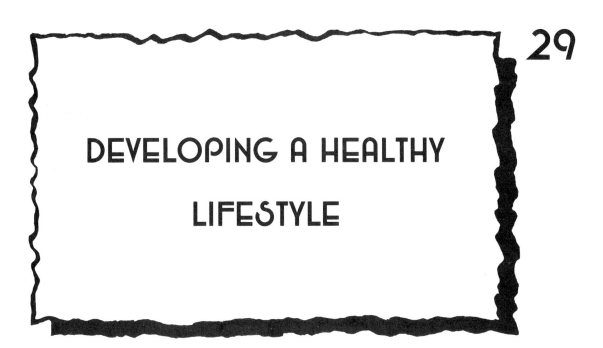

29

DEVELOPING A HEALTHY LIFESTYLE

To be an effective and resourceful coper, you need more than a collection of stress management strategies. In this chapter we will consider five lifestyle *risk behaviors* that can contribute to stress and illness: lack of exercise, poor nutrition, smoking, alcohol abuse, and drug abuse. These behaviors are closely linked to stress in a variety of ways. They can increase your vulnerability. They are often self-defeating attempts to defend against, or avoid confronting, stress situations. The stress management approaches presented in this book can be a powerful part of programs designed to reduce risk behaviors. And reducing a risk behavior can enhance your ability to cope.

Exercise

Exercise is clearly healthy. The list of benefits could fill pages and includes: improving the lungs, heart, and circulatory system; delaying the degenerative effects of aging; helping to maintain normal blood pressure; producing quicker recovery time from stress; improving posture, endurance, and physical appearance; and helping to maintain ideal weight. In fact, a major study of thousands of middle-aged men showed clearly the payoffs of exercise (Paffenberger et al. 1984). Moderate exercisers lived longer, even when the effects of hypertension, obesity, and cigarette smoking were factored out.

Unfortunately, most Americans who resolve to get regular exercise quit within six months (Dishman, 1982). And, in spite of a well-documented explosion of interest in fitness, few people exercise sufficiently or regularly enough to benefit them (Genest & Genest, 1987). However, people are most likely to continue to exercise if their programs can be easily woven into their daily routines and if exercise is done with others. Indeed, businesses are beginning to introduce exercise programs at the workplace for just this reason.

An effective exercise program should involve from 15 to 60 minutes of fairly intense, continuous aerobic exercise three to five times a week (American College of Sports Medicine, 1978). Aerobic exercise includes any form of physical activity that significantly increases heart, breathing, and metabolic rate. Examples include jogging, swimming, aerobic dancing, jumping rope, continuous bicycling, cross-country skiing, and playing tennis or racketball. Lifting weights and playing golf or baseball are not aerobic exercises.

Whatever the activity, a quality program should include a number of features:

It should be supervised by a qualified professional.

If you are over 35, or have any health concern, it is important to obtain a physical before beginning (and inform your physician of your decision to start exercising).

A good program should be tailored to your strengths and weaknesses, and be challenging without subjecting your body to physical risk.

Training should include five to ten minutes of mild warm-up activity before exercise and an equal period of mild cool-down activity after exercise.

Exercises should gradually increase in difficulty, starting in the first weeks with those that are relatively easy for you.

Watch out for overtraining symptoms, such as fatigue, chronic depression, or accelerated or uneven heart rate.

Try not to let exercise be a stress enhancer for you. Check your thoughts during exercise to see if they are useful and rational (Chapters 6 through 8).

In addition, a number of factors may help you adhere to an exercise program (Oldridge, 1984). It is important to monitor your progress (number of exercises completed, changes in weight or heart rate) on a daily basis. Observable signs of success can do much to keep you exercising. In addition, reward yourself for exercising by using the contracting ideas suggested throughout this book. Identify and eliminate environmental stimuli likely to distract you from your exercise (walking next to a restaurant on the way home or exercising at a time when friends are likely to call). Finally, exercise with others who can give you social support for continuing; if you exercise alone, let others know about your commitment.

In considering exercise, think of what you already do and what you would like to do. Most exercise can be divided into four groups: calisthenics, or stretching exercises, designed to increase flexibility; isotonics, which involve pushing and lifting heavy objects (weight lifting); isometrics, which involve contraction of the muscles without body movement (making a fist, pushing both hands together, pushing against a wall); and aerobics (which we will explain). Table 29-1 offers a useful chart of activities, how much energy they consume, advantages, and disadvantages.

Aerobic exercise may have particular value for managing stress. Aerobic exercise puts additional demands on the heart, making it pump more. As a result, heart rate becomes more efficient. In addition, aerobic exercise increases muscle strength and endurance as well as lung capacity, strengthens bones, and improves cholesterol level.

To work, an aerobic exercise must increase heartbeat to 50 percent (if you are a beginner) or even 80 percent (if you are in condition) of its maximal rate. Here is how you compute your target heart rate. Subtract your age from 226 (if you are male) and 220 (if you are female). This is your maximal heart

TABLE 29-1 Activity Chart

Activity	*Energy Use**	*Advantages*	*Possible Disadvantages***
Walking	+ +	No cost, no equipment, no special facilities. Everyone can participate. Year-round activity	Time commitment, must walk fast for conditioning effect.
Jogging (less than five miles per hour)	+ + +	Promotes weight loss, leg strength, cardiovascular endurance. No special facilities.	May be hard on knees and other joints. Must have physical checkup, proper shoes.
Running (more than five miles per hour)	+ + + +	Promotes weight loss, cardiovascular conditioning, and well-being.	Must have physical checkup, good shoes. Can be hard on joints.
Dancing (Disco, other fast dances)	+ + +	Promotes weight control, total-body conditioning, esp. aerobic dancing (doing cardiovascular exercises to music). Year-round activity.	Must be brisk for conditioning. Requires coordination, rhythm for set dance patterns. May be hard on joints.
Biking	+ + +	Good cardiovascular conditioning, promotes weight control, easier on joints than walking, jogging, running. Energy-saving transportation.	Danger from autos, cost of bike, requires learned skill.
Alpine skiing	+ + +	Promotes total body conditioning, esp. legs. Enjoyable, apt to promote well-being.	Requires learned skill, expensive equipment. Can be dangerous, esp. if not in condition, from falls, cold weather, and altitude. Seasonal.
Cross-country skiing	+ + + +	Excellent for cardiovascular conditioning, total-body fitness. Little jar to body joints. Apt to promote well-being.	Requires some learned skill, special equipment. Cold and altitude may be a negative factor. Seasonal.
Swimming	+ + +	Excellent for cardiovascular conditioning and muscle toning. No jar to joints.	Requires some skill, pool, minimum cost of swimsuit.
Racket sports (tennis, squash, racketball)	+ + +(+)	Excellent total-body conditioner if fast game is played. Promotes weight loss.	Requires learned skill, special equipment and facilities. Must play at high level for conditioning effect.
Golf (walk, carry own clubs)	+ +	Enjoyable and relaxing if not self-critical. Some of the same benefits as walking.	Requires learned skill, special equipment. Walking briskly without intermittent stops is a better conditioner.
Bowling	+	Relaxing and enjoyable if not self-critical. Better than just sitting.	Almost no conditioning effect. Requires learned skill and special equipment. Not recommended as treatment or preventive relaxation technique.

(*continued*)

TABLE 29-1 (Continued)

Activity	Energy Use*	Advantages	Possible Disadvantages**
Calisthenics	+ +	Brisk, total-body exercises have conditioning value, esp. muscle toning. No cost, little or no equipment. Year-round activity.	May exacerbate existing muscle problems. Tendency to overdo initially.
Weight lifting	+ +	Increases strength, improves physique and may improve self-image. Can improve cardiovascular efficiency by lifting lighter weights for greater repetitions or by circuit training.	Requires special equipment. Some risk of muscular injury unless properly trained and prudently utilized.

*All energy use, of course, depends on the intensity at which one pursues the activity, so only a relative rating system is used here. One "+" denotes least strenuous activity and minimal energy use, while four "+" signs denotes highest energy use.

**A possible disadvantage in most of these activities is high-level, ego-involved competition.

Source: Adapted by permission from: Girdango/Everly/Dusek, *Controlling Stress and Tension: A Holistic Approach*, 3e, © 1990, pp. 268–269. Reprinted by permission of Prentice Hall, Englewood Cliffs, NJ.

rate. Then multiply it by 50%, 60%, 70%, or 80%, depending on your condition (and doctor's advice). The resulting number is your target heart rate. Take your rate by using an inexpensive pulse monitor available from most exercise or biking stores. You can also gently press the fingers of your left hand on the inside of your right wrist. It is often best to have someone else show you how to do this. Count your heart beat for 30 seconds. Then multiply your count by 2 to get your heart rate per minute. When taking your heart rate during exercise, stop and immediately take a measure.

An aerobic program can be completed in fifteen or twenty minutes a day, three days a week. If you are out of shape, start with shorter periods, such as five or ten minutes a day.

Nutrition

Good nutrition is obviously important. But the food we eat can also have an impact our response to stress. For example:

- Caffeine increases metabolic rate and the secretion of stress hormones.
- Under stress, our body is more likely to use up B and C vitamins.
- High sugar intake can contribute to hypoglycemia, a condition that often produces stresslike symptoms of irritability, anxiety, and fatigue.
- Too much sodium contributes to high blood pressure, also associated with stress.

Perhaps the most important dietary advice is to:

- Eat a balance and variety of foods
- Maintain your ideal body weight
- Avoid fats
- Eat whole, unprocessed foods
- Avoid sugar
- Avoid salt and sodium

- Avoid alcohol
- Avoid caffeine

Obesity Obesity is a risk factor in and of itself, and it contributes to other risk factors such as high blood pressure. Specifically, obesity has been associated with atherosclerosis (hardening of the arteries), high blood pressure, some forms of cancer, kidney disease, arthritis, and gall bladder disease. In addition, obesity makes surgery and childbearing more dangerous. Unfortunately, many people are overweight; approximately 14 percent of adult men and 24 percent of adult women in the United States are obese, that is, at least 20 percent overweight (Stunkard, 1975).

More people are treated for obesity than for all other risk behaviors combined (Stunkard, 1979). Generally, there are five approaches to weight loss (Straw, 1983; Wilson, 1984). *Dieting* is the most common approach and typically involves becoming educated about the basics of good nutrition. Unfortunately, dieting is a necessary but insufficient factor in lasting weight loss. *Fasting* involves severely restricting food intake over several days. Although this approach can quickly produce dramatic weight losses, fasting cannot continue without injuring health. Unless a fast is followed by a quality maintenance program, pounds quickly return. It should be noted that fasting is potentially dangerous and must also be accompanied by medical supervision. *Appetite-suppression drugs* may help weight loss initially, but they have side effects and cannot be taken for long periods of time. In rare cases, *surgical intervention* involving bypassing part of the small intestine or reducing the size of the stomach has been used to reduce caloric intake. Results are promising, but the medical risks can be severe.

Behavior modification, combined with dieting, exercise, and possibly fasting, is a particularly promising approach to treating obesity. Such programs treat loss of weight as a complex undertaking involving graduated steps. Important components include:

Determining and eliminating environmental stimulus cues that suggest or trigger eating (keeping food out in the open, spending time with friends who are always snacking, and shopping for food without a list);

Confining eating to certain times and places;

Gaining control over the process of eating (by slowly chewing food, and holding down utensils until food is swallowed);

Keeping careful records of food intake, and rewarding yourself for success;

Countering irrational and self-defeating thoughts and beliefs that can interfere with maintaining a weight loss program;

Using booster sessions to deal with problems that arise in maintaining ideal weight; and involving all members of the family

Combination behavioral approaches to weight loss have shown modest success. Participants can lose a pound or two per week for up to 20 weeks, and the losses are often maintained. Such programs show lower dropout rates and produce fewer side effects. (Brownell, 1982 & Stunkard, 1979).

We have provided some simple initial guidelines for exercise and good nutrition. However, the following risk behaviors, although stress-related, clearly require professional help. I will describe the types of professional programs now available. If you need help, check your local hospital, mental health clinic, or university for programs that are available in your area.

Smoking

Cigarette smoking is the largest preventable cause of death in the United States. Most people are familiar with the risks. Smokers are twice as likely to die from heart disease than nonsmokers. Smoking causes lung cancer, cancer of the mouth, and cancer of the urinary bladder. Indeed, smoking is a serious problem, associated with one in every four American deaths (Warner, 1986).

It is extremely difficult to stop smoking. Silvan Tomkins (1966,1968) has suggested four reasons for this. People smoke for pleasurable stimulation, habit, and psychological dependence on its ability to ease negative emotions such as anger and fear. Smoking is also used to reduce stress; indeed, heavy smokers have a much lower tolerance for stress when then quit (increasing their motivation to continue). In addition to these psychological factors, nicotine is physically addicting. The moment smoke enters the mouth (even before it reaches the lungs), nicotine is transmitted by the blood and to the brain. Here, it activates both the brain and sympathetic nervous system, arousing the body, producing pleasurable effects.

Given the severity of the problem, it is not surprising that a large number of treatments have evolved for stopping smoking. *Aversion therapy* involves pairing smoking with an unpleasant stimulus, such as an electric shock or an imagined aversive scene. Variations of this approach include focused smoking, in which the smoker deliberately attends to the unpleasant aspects of smoking (burning sensations, smell), and rapid smoking, in which the smoker rapidly and continuously smokes a large number of cigarettes. Such approaches are used less now because of potential health risks, particularly for heart patients.

Stimulus control strategies such as those applied in treating obesity involve determining and eliminating environmental stimuli that suggest and trigger smoking (smoking with friends and leaving cigarettes laying around the house). A novel stimulus approach involves carrying a buzzer timed to permit smoking at predetermined intervals (thereby removing environmental stimuli as a smoking trigger). Through *response substitution*, a smoker replaces smoking with a behavior incompatible with smoking (chewing gum right after breakfast). *Contingency contracts* involve committing oneself to precise smoking reduction goals, and rewarding oneself for goals achieved. *Fading* approaches involve changing cigarette brands weekly to ones containing less tar and nicotine. *Pharmacological* approaches involve chewing special nicotine gum to break the dependency on cigarettes for nicotine. A variety of *follow-up* strategies are designed to enhance long-term cessation of smoking. These include buddy systems and follow-up calls from friends with whom you have made arrangements to monitor your progress. Even admonitions from a physician can be a useful form of follow-up.

Many have concluded (Benfari, Ockene, & McIntyre, 1982; Leventhal & Cleary, 1980) that most treatments for smoking are initially quite successful (with success rates as high as 90 percent). However, dropout rates are high and improvements short-lived. After six months to a year, only 10 to 25 percent of those treated remain nonsmokers. And virtually all approaches are about equally effective, although combination approaches appear to have somewhat greater impact. Yet the statistics provide an element of hope. Since 1964, over 30 million Americans have stopped smoking (United States Public Health Service, Surgeon General's Report, 1982). It is quite possible that those who quit make multiple attempts. The first may well be unsuccessful. But as additional programs are attempted, new skills are acquired. Eventually, the smoker may acquire sufficient motivation and skill to stop for good (Schachter, 1982). Such attempts appear even more likely to be successful if combined with comprehensive smoking control programs at work. Here peer support, financial incentives, and a sense of healthy competition combine to enhance attempts to quit (Stachnik & Stoffelmayr, 1983).

Alcohol Abuse

The President's Commission on Mental Health (1978) defines an alcoholic as a person whose drinking problem impairs life adjustment in terms of health, personal relationships, and/or occupational functioning. From 10 to 15 million adult Americans are problem drinkers. The costs to health are severe. Alcohol consumption has been linked to cirrhosis of the liver, cancer, suicide, high blood pressure, and brain damage. Nearly half of highway fatalities are linked to alcohol. The life span of the average alcoholic is about 12 years shorter than the nonalcoholic, and alcohol ranks as the third major cause of death in America.

At one time alcoholics were institutionalized, an approach now considered unnecessary (Miller & Hester, 1985). As with obesity and smoking, a multifaceted treatment appears to be most effective. Generally, treatment goals include: physical rehabilitation, control over drinking, and development of skills to cope with life without alcohol.

For acute intoxication, the initial treatment goal is detoxification (elimination of alcohol from the blood, minimizing potentially dangerous withdrawal symptoms), and physical rehabilitation.

Detoxification alone is not a long-term solution. Long-term treatment can involve a variety of strategies. Often disulfiram (Antabuse) is prescribed. This drug creates very uncomfortable effects whenever one drinks even the smallest amount of alcohol. Disulfiram can be useful for helping the alcoholic break a drinking cycle before beginning a broader-based treatment. At times, other aversive stimuli (noxious images, electric shock) are paired with drinking.

A substantial number of behavioral approaches are often used to treat alcoholism. These include: controlling stimuli (removing suggestive and tempting environmental cues, such as keeping alcohol in the refrigerator or driving home past taverns); teaching behaviors incompatible with drinking (consuming coffee or soft drinks at a party); careful monitoring of success at abstaining; and contracting for and rewarding abstinence. In addition, alcoholics are often enrolled in group therapy in which they are forced to assess their problems, avoidance strategies, and coping options. Such treatment may involve spouses and children.

Alcoholics Anonymous (AA) is one extremely popular self-help treatment approach. Started in 1935, AA now claims over one million members. AA is primarily a nonprofessional counseling and support program. Its basic philosophy is that people who abuse alcohol are alcoholics for life, even if they never take another drink. Taking just one drink after stopping is viewed as enough to trigger a drinking binge. The AA philosophy has nonsectarian spiritual roots; one of its 12 steps states that the alcoholic must "admit to God, to ourselves, and to another human being the exact nature of our wrongs." Most attend about four AA meetings a week. These meetings include a variety of social activities, discussion of problems and successes, and group support.

AA claims that two out of three participants succeed in stopping drinking. Indeed, one authorized study found a 75 percent success rate (Robinson, 1979). However, little research has been conducted on AA, partly because members must maintain anonymity. It is known that many drop out of the program. In addition, some studies show AA to be somewhat less effective than professional approaches (Brandsma, Maultsby, & Welsh, 1980). At the very least, AA may be appropriate for those who feel comfortable with its spiritual philosophy.

What makes an alcoholism treatment program successful? A number of factors appear to be important. First, the alcoholic must be treated early. In addition, it is important to alter the entire environment of the alcoholic, including family and work. Enlisting support from family, friends, and co-workers can enhance success. Follow-up should be included in which success is monitored. And, as we have noted, combination treatment approaches are more effective than single methods of treatment.

One highly emotional issue is the debate over acceptability of controlled, moderate drinking as opposed to total abstinence as a treatment goal. At the very least, controlled drinking is not a wise option for the long-term alcoholic. Those most likely to succeed appear to be young and socially stable (married and employed), to have a brief history of alcohol abuse without serious withdrawal symptoms, and to prefer drinking in moderation (Peele, 1984).

Substance Abuse

Apart from alcohol, the most widely abused drugs in America are: *narcotics* (opium, codeine, and heroin), *sedatives* (barbiturates), *stimulants* (cocaine and amphetamines), *anti-anxiety drugs* (meprobamates and minor tranquilizers), and *hallucinogens* (marijuana, LSD, mescaline, and PCP). It is estimated that more than three million Americans suffer from drug abuse or dependency (Cohen, 1986).

Unfortunately, the effects of drug abuse are not as well documented as those of cigarette and alcohol abuse or lack of exercise and obesity. This is because drug abuse is a relatively recent problem and, because of severe criminal sanctions, many who use drugs are reluctant to participate in studies. However, a few facts are known. Use of heroin is perhaps the most serious problem. Its costs include addiction, death, disability, family disruption, and increased crime. Smoking marijuana damages lungs and is implicated in many accidents. Cocaine can trigger cardiac arrhythmia, lead to heart attacks, destroy liver cells, and cause brain seizures. Excessive use of barbiturates can slow speech, impair mental functioning, cause mood shifts, impair motor coordination, trigger depression, and eventually may cause brain damage. Stimulants can trigger high blood pressure (possibly leading to death), brain damage, as well as psychotic reactions. Finally, hallucinogens can trigger adverse emotional reactions.

Drug abuse is often a deeply entrenched problem resistant to treatment, particularly if addiction is involved. The little research that has been conducted suggests, once again, that it appears useful to start with detoxification and then combine a variety of behavioral and cognitive methods, similar to what is often used for treating alcoholism. Then, for narcotic addiction, certain chemical agents can effectively block the euphoric effects of heroin, morphine, and codeine. Methadone, the most widely used treatment, can be very effective in reducing an addict's need for opiates (Bardo & Risner, 1985; Callahan, 1980).

30

COPING CREATIVELY

The key to stress management is not so much knowing a few specific techniques as it is knowing how to experiment and explore. My goal has been to teach the skills basic to optimism, the skills for finding tools, trying them out, assessing which work and do not work, and even letting go of those that are not helpful. These are the skills of creative coping, the skills basic to healthy optimism.

In this chapter we take a closer look at creative coping. An excellent way of doing this is in the context of a coping team. Here members can share tools they have found or invented. The formula we have used throughout this book works with any tool you find: WARNING SIGN/CRITICAL MOMENT → COPE → REWARD We begin with examples of creative coping unearthed by members of coping teams I have run.

Examples of Creative Coping

Humor Humor can be a tool for dealing with stress (Nezu, Nezu, & Blissett, 1988). If you think about this seriously, the reasons are clear. Humor helps us see things in perspective and avoid stressful thinking (Chapters 6 and 7). It is hard to imagine genuinely laughing at the absurdity of a situation while thinking "this is the end of the world." A good sense of humor is enjoyed by others, increasing future support we can get from them in return. Seeing the humor of a situation involves taking an active stance towards the world rather than giving up. You are choosing to see the world on your terms, and you see it for the joke it really is.

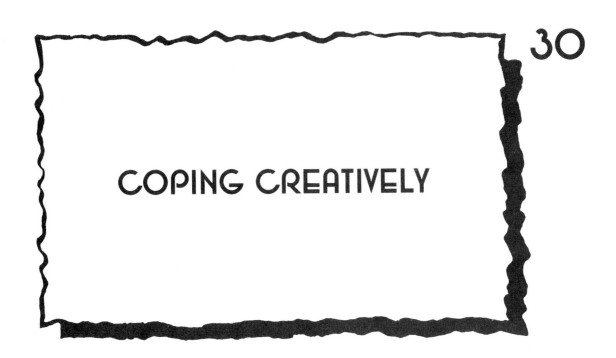

One coping team member discovered some hints for humor in a popular book on stress (Faelten & Diamond, 1988). Here are the hints she found useful:

- Remind myself to have fun.
- Keep a "silly scrapbook" in which I collect jokes, cartoons, and amusing photos.
- Take an occasional laugh break. Bring something funny to work or to church.
- Lighten up. Think how my favorite comedian would handle a stressful situation.
- I think of a stressful situation as if it were an awful episode of some comedy show. I sit back in amazement at how bad it gets.
- Spend time with some people I find amusing.

Journal Writing

Opening up to another person is the secret of psychotherapy. Painful and hidden feelings are brought out into the air and become less disturbing. This desensitizing process has been known for years by therapists. But recently, research suggests that at least some value can come from opening up in journal writing. Here is a discovery one coping team member made:

> Recently I read a book, *Opening Up*, by James Pennebacker (1990) that suggested that confiding in others is a useful and powerful way of coping with stress. He even showed research showing the effect of confiding on physical stress. He suggested one technique, writing your feelings down. I tried it, and it works. Here's what I did. It wasn't necessary for me to write about the most serious traumas. I started by writing about issues that were important to me at the time. I explored both the specifics of what happened, and my feelings about it. I wrote continuously, not worrying at all about grammar or spelling. If I ran out of things to write, I simply repeated. I made sure my writing was absolutely anonymous, and didn't show it to anyone. At first, I burned my journal pages. Later I kept them. Because no one would ever see what I was writing, I could be completely honest, and let down all my defenses.
>
> Of course, there were some problems in this approach. At first I found I was at times using writing as a substitute for effective action. It was more helpful to write about my feelings and reactions to making sincere and active attempts at coping. I had to take care not to make my writing an intellectual exercise, to show how intelligent I was. Throwing my writing away helped cure that. At times my writing became just a form of uncensored complaining, whining, and self-absorption. But, all told, the pluses outweighed the minuses. I like writing. I helps me sort out my ideas. Often, when I start writing, I am not at all sure what will come out.

Pets

A creative search for coping options does not always require scientific validation. Frankly, I think there will always be more promising coping options than researchers could ever hope to study. Once again, the key is knowing how to experiment. This was demonstrated by one coping team member, a struggling and not particularly successful writer.

> I have a gentle, brown Burmese cat whose name is Moco. Ordinarily I don't get sentimental about animals, but one day Moco taught me a little lesson about coping. I was buried in an urgent and complicated writing project. My mind wandered from one idea to the next. I felt scattered and unfocused. Then, suddenly, Moco jumped on my computer keyboard and

stared directly in my eyes. I was startled out of my confusion. She then walked away, very slowly, very simply, but with clear determination. "Ah, a lesson on living in the moment," I thought. "Step slowly and simply, one problem at a time." I then looked at the computer screen. One small leap had generated a truly spectacular array of "X's" and "Z's." "Ah, how kind. She even gives me a chance to try out this lesson in coping."

Creative Coping and Critical Thinking

Any explorer of coping faces a harsh and threatening world. Although there are indeed many techniques worth trying, there are also many worth ignoring. How can you tell the difference? First, I believe techniques you have invented on your own, if they are safe, are worth trying out. However, I am more concerned about fancy looking and often expensive gizmos, rituals, and treatments that frequently appear in the popular press. These are often promoted with some vigor as "proven effective," and often have hidden costs. At the very least, they can waste valuable time that might be spent learning good coping skills. But how can you tell the fads, frauds, and fictions? I believe that a sensible consumer of stress management should at least be aware of the three "P's" of poor science: Placebos, Pseudoscience, and the P.T. Barnum Effect.

Placebos

The placebo is a claimed medical treatment that has no specific reason for working. It is, in other words, the proverbial "sugar pill." What makes a placebo work is the simple belief that the treatment is legitimate.

It is important to recognize that placebos are a standard part of medical research. The reason for this may surprise you: for almost any disorder, a certain number of individuals will recover simply because of their belief that a treatment will work. For example, in a typical study on pain, about a quarter will benefit from an actual pain treatment, such as aspirin. Almost an equal number will benefit from a fake treatment, a sugar pill described as "aspirin." A general rule of thumb is that, as the severity of a disorder increases, the number of "placebo responders" decreases; relative few (although some!) cancer and heart patients benefit from placebos. In contrast, for milder disorders, especially those in which anxiety is the main problem, placebos are more effective. Whatever the disorder, an experimental treatment is not considered acceptable unless it works better than a placebo. In other words, a valid medical treatment must do a better job than simple faith in a treatment.

On one hand, the placebo is impressive proof of the powers of the human mind. Think of it—simple belief can be enough to reduce some symptoms. Indeed, many of the approaches to stress management presented in this book make use of this powerful "belief factor." However, a placebo can also be a tricky deception, a fake treatment claimed to do more than it actually can.

How can you tell if you are getting a placebo? One way is to take a close look at the treatment itself. Research reveals an interesting set of factors that make placebos work. Of course, the recipient must believe in the treatment. If you think your treatment is a fake, it is much less likely to work. Second, the person who *gives* the treatment must also believe in it. If two nurses give their patients identical placebos, and one believes the treatment to be an actual painkiller, the patients of this nurse will actually do better. Indeed, the nurse need not say a thing to the patients; belief alone can be manifest by subtle body cues.

If a "placebo," or fake treatment, is *complicated* and *sophisticated*, it is more likely to work. Imagine two black boxes, both claimed to cure headaches. Add to one an impressive array of wires, lights, dials, and perhaps even a TV monitor, and it will have a greater placebo effect. Its sheer complexity and sophistication will have a greater impact on headaches. Such complexity and sophistication need not be restricted to equipment. Any simple procedure can be made complex. For example, if you wish to claim the power of curing headaches by gently touching a patient's forehead, be sure to make it an impressive ritual. You might chant a variety of obscure phrases, pace around the patient a few times, and close your eyes tightly. Once again, complicated and sophisticated placebos work better.

In addition, if a placebo is accompanied by a complicated, plausible *explanation* of why it should work, it will work better. Indeed, the explanation may be pure nonsense—but if it sounds good, and complicated, that is all that is needed. Take our worthless headache treatment box in the preceding example. Effectiveness can be boosted considerably by adding an impressive rationale. You might say, for example:

> This box detects subtle brain wave patterns that cause headaches. Through a complex computer-filtering process, brainwaves are deprogrammed for the component responsible for the headache, and then subliminally fed back to you visually by means of this TV screen. The headache-free brainwaves gradually replace the headache waves and you are cured.

Of course, this is sheer nonsense. But it sounds good, and it is complicated—and that is enough to make a placebo work better.

Finally, good placebos have side effects. It is indeed true that bitter medicine is better. If a patient is presented with believable (although perfectly false) evidence of efficacy, a placebo is more likely to work. This evidence can simply be the unpleasantness of the treatment. It can be contrived feedback from fake medical equipment. Even spontaneous reactions by a patient ("This treatment is so long . . . I'm feeling tired and bored.") can be reinterpreted as signs of effectiveness ("Good! Boredom and fatigue are signs that the treatment is working.")

Illegitimate placebos, not used in medical research, are often imposed upon an unsuspecting public. Perhaps the most dramatic and gruesome in recent years was psychic surgery. In the mid-1960s and 1970s psychic surgeons in the Philippines claimed the ability to insert their hands into a patient's body and perform "surgery" without making any kind of incision. During surgery, the psychic's hand would seem to disappear into the patient's belly. A pool of blood would appear. After a few minutes, the psychic would dramatically pull out a bloody organ, ulcer, or diseased tumor. Remarkably, after surgery not the slightest mark would be found on the patient—a rather impressive medical miracle.

Psychic surgery patients frequently claimed to feel much better, and more than a few members of the news media were impressed. Indeed, tens of thousands of people made the pilgrimage to the Philippines for treatment. Unfortunately, psychic surgery was nothing more than an elaborate deception, and their placebo-generated cures were short-lived (Nolen, 1974). What in fact happened is an excellent illustration of the placebo-boosting qualities we have just described. First, the typical patient believed deeply in the reality of psychic surgery, often enough to travel thousands of miles. And the procedure was indeed sophisticated. The surgeon hid in his or her hand, or in a hollow fake thumb, blood and animal tissue. After the complex ritual of rubbing and probing the patient's abdomen (often so vigorously that it appeared the hand was entering the abdomen), the bloody contents were discharged. Observers were convinced the surgery was a success. The patient saw objective evidence of surgery. And the placebo worked.

Pseudoscience

Psychic surgery is perhaps one of the more peculiar blends of placebos and pseudoscience. Pure forms of pseudoscience often find their way into popular literature on stress management. As we shall see, often their persuasiveness is enhanced by the same "placebo-making" characteristics that can increase the impact of sugar pills. Terence Hines (1988) has written an important textbook, *Pseudoscience and the Paranormal*, which gives us many insights about the nature of pseudoscience. Perhaps the most revealing characteristic of pseudoscience is the "irrefutable hypothesis." Science progresses only when false hypotheses are discovered to be in error. Consider where we would be today if we still accepted the hypothesis that the earth is flat. Evidence eventually proved this notion wrong; it was a refutable hypothesis. However, consider another hypothesis, one that might be offered by, say, a schizophrenic patient: "I can read all of your unconscious thoughts, all the hidden ideas you are unaware of." How could you possibly prove this notion wrong? Each time you say "No, you're wrong, I wasn't thinking that," the patient could simply respond, "Yes, you were. You were thinking it unconsciously!" The patient has an irrefutable hypothesis; it cannot be disproved. Irrefutable hypotheses are often found in popularized presentations of stress management techniques.

Imagine that a stress management instructor informs you that: "Meditation cures stress. If meditation didn't cure your stress, you didn't practice it long (or effortfully) enough." Notice how this claim is irrefutable. No matter how long or diligently you practice meditation, the failure of the technique for you is not evidence for the meditation's ineffectiveness. One could still claim you should have practiced longer or with more concentration.

In addition, proponents of pseudoscience characteristically have very low standards for evaluating their evidence. I remember one example vividly. Years ago, I was asked to appear on a radio show to discuss stress. The moderator asked my opinion of a new stress management device called the Ultimo Chair. Developed by a philosophy professor, this titanium-framed device actually looked like a Buck Rogers style of lawn chair. Wires sprouted ominously out of every joint. Everything connected to an impressive electrical gadget in the center. According to the inventor, subtle bodily signals could be picked up by the chair and transmitted to a computer and music amplifier. Then, depending on your level of stress, various violin melodies would play, the pace and intensity determined by your level of tension.

I asked about the effectiveness of the Ultimo Chair. The moderator assured me that its developer had tried it out on a few friends, and they felt it worked wonderfully. Unfortunately, as near as I could tell, this testing and his background in philosophy were the extent of the evidence for the chair's effectiveness. Yet, its developer was willing to sell the device nationally for nearly $1,000!

Although proponents of pseudoscience have very low standards for evaluating their own claims, their standards for critics are impossibly high. Often this is their rule: "What I claim is true, unless you can disprove every case." Take this example: I announce that Santa Claus really exists. If you discover that last year's Christmas present really came from your parents, I simply state that, to disprove my claim, you have to prove that *every* Christmas present in the world did not come from Santa. Obviously, you cannot sneak into every household the night before Christmas to show that I am wrong. I am asking too much; indeed, it is not your responsibility to disprove anything. Since I am making the extraordinary claim (that Santa exists), it is my job to find evidence to support this claim. The burden of proof rests squarely on the person making the claim.

While the developer of the Ultimo Chair seemed to have very low standards for evidence supporting the effectiveness of his invention, his standards for possible conflicting evidence were extremely high. The radio moderator had asked prior to the show if he would mind appearing with me on a program to discuss stress management. The inventor objected vehemently, claiming that, since I was a professional psychologist, I could hardly be expected to evaluate his device objectively; my having published several scientific books and articles seemed to make little difference. His standards for others scientific claims appeared to be higher than for himself.

P. T. Barnum Techniques

Many proponents of pseudoscientific approaches to stress management have subtle and clever ways of impressing and moving their customers. These manipulations are referred to here as "P. T. Barnum techniques," named after the famous (and somewhat notorious) circus showman noted for his wise but cynical observation, "There's a sucker born every minute."

P. T. Barnum techniques can perhaps be most clearly seen in the application of astrology. In spite of about 50 well-designed studies, there is absolutely no scientific evidence for astrology (Hines, 1988). However, many astrologers claim that customers find astrological interpretations useful for stress management. Of course, many superstitions can be useful: a child may find clutching a security blanket or rabbit's foot a helpful way of confronting a trip to the dentist. More seriously, the capacity of humans for self-deception and suggestion is, if you will, astronomical. Studies have shown that astrological interpretations:

1. Are sufficiently general to be true for nearly everyone. (Astrologer: "You may have some sexual concerns; you are more anxious at times than you desire; you worry about a close friend; you are more creative than you think." Customer: "Wow! How did you know that?")
2. Contain specific interpretations that can be subtly altered and reinterpreted to fit the customer. (Astrologer: "You are sad over the death of your mother." Customer: "But my mother is still alive." Astrologer: "Ah yes, of course, your sadness is over a future death of someone close to you.")

TABLE 30-1 Popular Examples of Pseudoscience

Astrology
Bermuda Triangle
Creationism
Crystals as Stress Management
Flying saucers
Krilian photography
"Moon madness"
Pyramid Power
Scientology
Shroud of Turin
Silva Mind Control
Subliminal Tapes as Cures for Stress
Transcendental Meditation

3. Contain so many details that nearly everyone will find some that fit, and forget those that do not. (Astrologer: "You are sociable, but at times shy; creative, but often stuck in a rut; calm, but aware of things that might make you anxious; intelligent, but at times annoyingly slow." Customer: "Amazing! How did know about my shyness?")
4. Are often based, not on a reading of a specific horoscope, but on the wealth of nonverbal cues presented by a client (body language, clothing, facial expression or jewelry). Such cues enable professional magicians (who claim no paranormal powers) to make impressively accurate "dry readings" of personality. (Astrologer, noting the customer's gold chain, expensive hair style, marriage ring, and facial scar: "You have done well in life, better than many. You are currently very close to someone, perhaps a marriage partner. However, I sense a recent tragedy." Customer: "Wow! You really read my mind!")

Such clever manipulations are not exclusive to astrology. A legion of popularized approaches to stress management have gained some credibility through the application of similar P. T. Barnum techniques.

Creative stress management holds the promise of opening many doors. However, it also poses many risks. The creative coper knows how to separate fact from fraud and substance from superstition.

31

GRASPING THE BIG PICTURE

We began this book with an observation. Effective coping is based on creative resourcefulness. One has at hand a world of coping resources. But such optimism can only go so far and fails to deal with two thorny questions: "Why?" and "What if?" Why manage stress in the first place? Why keep on going when coping fails? At first, the answer may seem obvious: to reduce the costs of stress, that is, to live longer, healthier, happier, and more productively. But then why are these important?

Furthermore, what if nothing works? What if our best efforts at coping are not enough to deal with the problems life presents? Unfortunately, life presents us with such dilemmas. Consider the cancer patient, for whom no pain management or coping strategy works, and constant pain is a reminder of sickness and death. Consider the burned-out factory worker who cannot leave or change a frustrating work environment, and whose sensitizing, monitoring style of handling frustration does not permit defensive avoidance.

And what do you do if, after *succeeding* in reducing the hassles of life and achieving comfort and success, you *still* feel frustrated and empty? What techniques are available for dealing with emptiness that follows successful coping? We could go on, but the point is that optimism and coping are not enough to prepare us for the truly troublesome problems of living.

From time to time, we have touched upon a possible answer. Earlier we saw that a relaxation philosophy helps extend the impact of a relaxation exercise. Albert Ellis and others have taught us that rational and productive beliefs and assumptions enable us to reduce stress. We saw that a thoughtful consideration of life's long-term priorities is essential to time management. Empathy and commitment to others build stress-buffering social supports. And the belief that stressors are ultimately problems to be solved or negotiated is fundamental to all the strategies in this book. All of these notions point to a deeper idea: our philosophies of life can form the foundation for optimism and coping.

The Coping Philosophy

I have a friend who seems to deal with stress particularly well. I always wanted to know his secret technique. One day I asked him, and his answer surprised me. Instead of describing a special exercise or strategy, he said:

> Life is a teacher and I am the student. This may seem like a strange idea, but it keeps me going. Sometimes I seem to do quite well. I deal with the problems at work, assertively negotiate problems with my supervisor and co-worker, and enjoy my family. However, rather than boast of my success, I treat my successes as lessons. The same is true for my frustrations. Those times when nothing seems to work, and hassles just don't go away, are also lessons. Put very simply, I have a particular philosophy of life, something that helps me make sense of it all. There are meanings and messages deeper than I can ever comprehend; I am here to experience and to learn.

What is interesting is that my friend did not describe a specific set of coping strategies. Instead, he shared his thoughts concerning the meanings of stress and coping. But his thinking represents more than rational or pragmatic thoughts. Indeed, it goes beyond a problem-solving attitude. What we see is evidence of a basic and encompassing personal coping philosophy.

A coping philosophy provides a context for coping. It reminds us of our resources, both visible and hidden. It tells us when action is or is not called for. It helps guide our choices when we are confused. It gives us courage to act, even when we may feel too comfortable, depressed, anxious, or irritated to do so. It tells us when sacrifice is needed, and when it is not. Finally, our coping philosophy gives us a reason to persevere in the face of relapse.

A coping philosophy must answer at least three basic questions: What do I believe in? What do I value? and What are my commitments? Our *beliefs* consist of our enduring thoughts about what is real and factual. What are the facts concerning ourselves, others, and the world? Examples include:

"The earth travels around the sun."

"Smoking is unhealthy."

"Assertive people have less stress."

"Relaxation reduces stress and tension."

Our *values* consist of what we think is important. For example:

"I want to live a long and healthy life."

"Friends are important to me."

"I want to be successful at work."

"I value doing my best."

Finally, our *commitments* represent what actions we have chosen to take. Examples include:

"I have decided to read and try this stress management book."

"I am committed to reducing my weight by cutting down on fats in my diet."

"I have decided to give generously to my church."

"I will spend at least one day a week with my family."

Obviously, not all beliefs, values, and commitments can be part of a coping philosophy. They must, once again, provide a context for coping—a reason to try, and a reason to go on living when we fail. They must point to resources we have, both seen and unseen. However, there is no single, correct coping philosophy. Part of the deeper process of learning to cope is deciding what you truly believe, value, and are committed to.

A Gallery of Philosophies

We conclude this book, not with a single philosophical vision, but with a gallery of visions which students, clients, and patients have shared with me over the years. I find something important happens when I listen openly and nonjudgmentally to someone's coping philosophy. I feel enriched. My own philosophy is challenged and deepened. Most important, I am prompted to look beyond my own narrow perspective and see the world with greater hope and optimism.

We begin with Raymond, who is a computer specialist. Raymond focuses on healthy living:

> My health is important to me. I can do many things to foster health. I believe in assertively stating what's on my mind. It's unhealthy to keep my feelings bottled in. I believe in systematically attempting to solve problems. It's unhealthy to let problems sit and fester. Work is healthy. Love and fun are healthy. The release of tension through daily meditation is healthy. And through healthy living, I believe something deeper happens. I work in harmony with those hidden biological forces in my brain that contribute to life and healing.

Josephine is not a particularly religious person. She does not belong to any organized church. However, her coping philosophy is clearly spiritual:

> I believe in a higher power, a deeper resource, an energy that is always there that underlies everything. What this resource is, I do not know. I do know that I can count on it. It gives answers. It supports me. It directs me. It gives me energy and courage. In fact, I experience it as the source of all that is beautiful and loving.

Richard is a writer. Like most writers, he experiences times of low productivity and times of inspiration. He has learned to cope with these shifts:

> Where do my ideas come from? I certainly cannot claim complete authorship. Often ideas come when I least expect them, and just as often, they do not come when I try my hardest to stir them up. I guess I have come to terms with my creative unconscious. I have learned to respect it

as the coauthor of my life. I do my part through hard work, study, living, and loving. And then I remain open to the unconscious resources that go beyond my efforts.

What is your coping philosophy? Many people have not thought through a complete answer. Indeed, a coping philosophy often grows in bits and pieces, often in response to life's challenges. It is at these times we come to terms with the three basic questions:

Belief Questions: "What is basically real and true about myself, others, and the world?"

"I have the ability to learn to cope."

"Poor problem-solving skills create stress."

"Stress and tension are unhealthy."

"Relaxation releases unhealthy tension."

"God has a plan for my life."

"My worries and concerns are the result of distorted thinking."

"Even failure can be a teacher."

Value Questions: "What is most important to me? Why is it important to learn effective coping and defense strategies? What remains important even when I fail?

"Love and compassion are most important to me."

"I want to reach my potential."

"God's plan is all that really counts."

"I can do without my possessions. They are not the most important thing."

"Some things are even more important than my deepest miseries."

Commitment Questions: "What am I willing to do in light of my beliefs and values? How am I willing to sacrifice time and effort?"

"I will devote time to practicing relaxation."

"I choose to be frank and honest whenever it is appropriate."

"I will take some risks in trying new coping solutions."

"Even if my stressful thinking seems true, I will look for ways I may be thinking in a self-defeating or irrational manner."

"God's will be done."

"I choose to treat stress as a problem to be solved."

A coping philosophy is not something chiseled in stone. It is always changing and growing. It is a product of courageously experimenting and trying out coping skills. And once formed, it becomes the firm ground on which a healthy optimism can flourish.

REFERENCES

American College of Sports Medicine. (1978). Position statement on the recommended quantity and quality of exercise for developing and maintaining fitness in healthy adults. *Medicine and Science in Sports, 10*, 7–10.

Antonovsky, A. (1979). *Health, stress, and coping.* San Francisco: Jossey-Bass.

Bandura, A. (1982). Self-efficacy mechanism in human agency. *American Psychologist, 37*, pp. 122–147.

Bandura, A. (1977). Self-efficacy: Toward a unifying theory of behavioral change. *Psychological Review, 84*, 191–215.

Bardo, M. T. & Risner, M. E. (1985). Biochemical substrates of drug abuse. In M. Galizio & S. A. Maisto (Eds.), *Determinants of substance abuse: Biological, psychological, and environmental factors.* New York: Plenum.

Beck, A. (1976). *Cognitive therapy and the emotional disorders.* New York: International Universities Press.

Beck, A. T. & Beamesderfer, A. (1974). Assessment of depression: The depression inventory. In P. Pichot (Ed.), *Modern problems in pharmacopsychiatry, vol 7.*

Beck, A., Rush, J., Hollon, S., & Shaw, B. (1979). *Cognitive therapy of depression.* New York: Guildford.

Beecher, H. K. (1959). *Measurement of subjective responses.* New York: Oxford University Press.

Benfari, R. C., Ockene, J. K., & McIntyre, K. M. (1982). Control of cigarette smoking from a psychological perspective. *Annual Review of Public Health, 3*, 101–128.

Borkovec, T. D. (1985). What's the use of worrying. *Psychology Today, 19*, 59–64.

Borkovec, T. D., Wilkinson, L., Folensbee, R., & Lerman, C. (1983). Stimulus control applications to the treatment of worry. *Behaviour Research and Therapy, 21*, 247–251.

Bower, S. A. & Bower, G. H. (1976). *Asserting Yourself.* Menlo Park, CA: Addison-Wesley.

Brandsma, J. M., Maultsby, M. C., & Welsh, R.J. (1980). *Outpatient treatment of alcoholism: A review and comparative study.* Baltimore: University Park Press.

Brownell, K. D. (1982). Obesity: Understanding and treating a serious, prevalent and refractory disorder. *Journal of Consulting and Clinical Psychology, 50*, 820–840.

Burns, D. D. (1989). *The feeling good handook.* New York: William Morrow & Company.

Callahan, E. J. (1980) Alternative strategies in the treatment of narcotic addiction: A review. In W. R. Miller (Ed.), *The addictive behaviors: Treatment of alcoholism, drug abuse, smoking, and obesity.* New York: Pergamon.

Cannon, W. B. (1929). *Bodily changes in pain, hunger, fear, and rage.* New York: Appleton.

Carver, C. S., Scheier, M. F., & Weintraub, J. K. (1989). Assessing coping strategies. A theoretically based approach. *Journal of Personality and Social Psychology, 56*, 267–283.

Cautela, J. R. & Wisocki, P. A. (1977). The thought-stopping procedure: Description, application, and learning theory interpretations. *Psychological Record, 1*, 255–264.

Cohen, S. (1986). Just say no. *Drug Abuse & Alcoholism Newsletter, 15*, No. 3.

Conger, J. C. & Farrell, A. D. (1981). Behavioral components of heterosocial skills. *Behavior Therapy, 12*, 41–55.

Cramer, K. D. (1990). *Staying on top when your world turns upside down.* New York: Viking.

Davis, M., Eshelman, E. R., & McKay, M. (1988). *The relaxation and stress reduction workbook.* Oakland, CA: New Harbinger.

Dembroski, T. M., MacDougall, J. M., Williams, B., & Haney, T. L. (1985). Components of Type A hostility and anger: Relationship to angiographic findings. *Psychosomatic Medicine, 47*, 219–233.

Derogatis, L. R. (1980). *The Derogatis Stress Profile.* Baltimore: Clinical Psychometric Research.

Dishman, R. K. (1982). Compliance/adherence in health-related exercise. *Health Psychology, 1*, 237–267.

D'Zurilla, T. J. (1986). *Problem-solving therapy: A social competence approach to clinical intervention.* New York: Springer Publishing Company.

Egan, G. (1976). *Interpersonal living: A skills/contract approach to human relations training in groups.* Pacific Grove CA: Brooks/Cole.

Egan, G. (1982). *The skilled helper.* Monterey, California: Brooks/Cole.

Egdahl, R. & Walsh, D. (1980) *Mental wellness programs for employees.* New York: Springer-Verlag.

Ellis, A. (1977). The basic clinical theory of rational-emotive therapy. In A. Ellis & R. Grieger (Eds.), *Handbook of rational-emotive therapy.* New York: Springer.

Ellis, A. & Harper, R. A. (1975). *A new guide to rational living.* Englewood Cliffs, NJ: Prentice-Hall.

Everly, G. S. & Girdano, D. A. (1980). *The stress mess solution: The causes of stress on the job.* Bowie, MD: Robert J. Brady.

Faelten, S. & Diamond, D. (1988). *Take control of your life: A complete guide to stress relief.* Emmaus, Pennsylvania: Rodale Press.

Freudenberger, H. J. (1980). *Burnout: The high cost of achievement.* Garden City, NY: Doubleday

Friedman, H. S. (Ed.) (1990). *Personality and disease.* New York: Wiley.

Friedman, M. & Rosenman, R. H. (1974). *Type A behavior and your heart.* New York: Knopf.

Gendlin, E. (1981). *Focusing.* New York: Bantam.

Genest, M. & Genest, S. (1987). *Psychology and health.* Champaign, IL: Research Press.

Girdano, D. A., Everly, G. S., Jr., & Dusek, D. E. (1990). *Controlling stress and tension.* Englewood Cliffs, NJ: Prentice Hall.

Glasgow, R. E. & Rosen, G. M. (1978). Behavioral bibliotherapy: A review of self-help behavior therapy manuals. *Psychological Bulletin, 85*, 1–23.

Glass, D. C. (1977). *Behavior patterns, stress, and coronary disease.* New York: Erlbaum.

Goldstein, A. P. & Keller, H. (1987). *Aggressive behavior: Assessment and intervention.* New York: Pergamon Press.

Goldstein, A. P., Sprafkin, R. P., & Gershaw, N. J. (1976). *Skill training for community living.* New York: Pergamon Press.

Goldstein, A. P. & Rosenbaum, A. (1982). *Agress-less.* Englewood Cliffs, NJ: Prentice-Hall.

Grasha, A. F. (1983). *Practical applications of psychology.* Boston, MA: Little, Brown and Company.

Greenberg, J. S. (1990). *Comprehensive stress management* (Third Edition). Dubuque, IA: Wm. C. Brown.

Greenwald, D. P. (1977). The behavioral assessment of differences in social skill and social anxiety in female college students. *Behavior Therapy, 8*, 925–937.

Haan, N. (1977). (Ed.) *Coping and defending: Processes of self-environment organization.* New York: Academic Press.

Haan, N. (1965). Coping and defense mechanisms related to personality inventories. *Journal of Consulting Psychology, 29*, 373–378.

Hanson, R. W. & Gerber, K. E. (1990). *Coping with chronic pain.* New York: Guilford.

Hines, T. (1988). *Pseudoscience and the Paranormal.* Buffalo, NY: Prometheus Books.

Holmes, T. H. & Rahe, R. H. (1967). The social readjustment rating scale. *Journal of Psychosomatic Research, 11*, 213–218.

Horowitz, M. J. (1976). *Stress response syndromes.* New York: Jason Aronson.

Hurrell, J. J., Jr., (1987). An overview of organizational stress and health. In L. R. Murphy & T. F. Schoenborn (Eds.), *Stress management in work settings.* Washington, DC.: National Institute for Occupational Safety and Health. (pp. 31–45).

Jackson, S. E., Schwab, R. L., & Schuler, R. S. (1986). Toward an understanding of the burnout phenomenon. *Journal of Applied Psychology, 71*, 630–640.

Jakubowski, P. & Lange, A. J. (1978). *The assertive option.* Champaign, IL: Research Press.

Jenkins, C. D., Rosenman, R. H., & Friedman, M. (1967). Development of an objective psychological test for the determination of the coronary-prone behavior pattern in employed men. *Journal of Chronic Diseases, 20*, 371–379.

Kanfer, F. H., & Gaelick-Buys, L. (1991). Self-management methods. In F. H. Kanfer & A. P. Goldstein (Eds.), *Helping people change.* New York: Pergamon Press. pp. 305–360.

Kanner, A. D., Coyne, J. C., Schaefer, C., & Lazarus, R. S. (1981). Comparison of two modes of stress measurement: Daily hassles and uplifts versus major life events. Journal of Behavioral Medicine, *4*, 1–39.

Kapleau, P. (1965). *The three pillars of Zen.* Boston: Beacon Press.

Kelly, G. A. (1955). *The psychology of personal constructs.* New York: W. W. Norton.

Kleinke, C. L, Meeker, F. B., & Staneski, R. A. (1986). Preference for opening lines: Comparing ratings by men and women. *Sex Roles, 15*, 585–600.

Kobasa, C. O., Maddi, S. R., & Courington, S. (1981). Personality and constitution as mediators in the stress-illness relationship. *Journal of Health and Social Behavior, 22*, 368–378.

Kukpke, T. E., Calhoun, K. S., & Hobbs, S. A. (1979). Selection of heterosocial skills, II. Experimental validity. *Behavior Therapy, 10*, 336–346.

Lakein, A. (1973). *How to get control of your time and your life.* New York: Signet.

Lazarus, R. S., & Folkman, S. (1984). *Stress, appraisal, and coping.* New York: Springer Publishing Company.

Leventhal, H. & Cleary, P. D. (1980). The smoking problem: A review of the research and theory in behavioral risk modification. *Psychological Bulletin, 88*, 370–405.

Luthe, W. (1965). *Autogenic training.* New York: Grune & Stratton.

MacDonald A. P. & Games, R. G. (1972). Ellis' irrational values. *Rational Living, 7*, 25–28.

Mackenzie, A. (1972). *The time trap.* New York: AMACOM.

Maslach, C. & Jackson, S. E. (1981). *The Maslach Burnout Inventory.* Palo Alto, CA: Consulting Psychologists Press.

McCarthy, M. (1988, April 7). Stressed employees look for relief in worker's compensation claims. *Wall Street Journal*, p. 34.

McMullin, R. E. (1986). *Handbook of cognitive therapy techniques.* New York: W. W. Norton.

Meichenbaum, D. (1985). *Stress inoculation training.* Elmsford, NY: Pergamon Press.

Melzack, R. & Wall, P. D. (1965). *Pain mechanisms: A new theory.* Science, 150, 971–979.

Melzack, R. & Wall, P. D. (1982). *The challenge of pain.* New York: Basic Books.

Miller, W. R. & Hester, R. K. (1985). Inpatient alcoholism treatment: Who benefits? *American Psychologist, 41*, 794–805.

Miller, S. Z. (1987). Monitoring and blunting: Validation of a questionnaire to assess styles of information seeking under threat. *Journal of Personality and Social Psychology, 52*, 345–353.

Nemeroff, C. J. & Karoly, P. (1991). Operant methods. In F. H. Kanfer & A. P. Goldstein (Eds.), *Helping People Change.* New York: Pergamon Press. pp. 122–160

Nezu, A. M., Nezu, C. M., & Blissett, S. E. (1988). Sense of humor as a moderator of the relation between stressful events and psychological distress: A prospective analysis. *Journal of Personality and Social Psychology, 54*, 520–525.

Nolen, W. (1974). *Healing: A Doctor in Search of a Miracle.* New York: Random House.
Novaco, R. W. (1975). *Anger control: The development and evaluation of an experimental treatment.* Lexington, MA: D. C. Heath.
Oldridge, N. B. (1984). Adherence to adult exercise fitness programs. In J. D. Matarazzo, S. M. Weiss, J. A. Herd, N. E. Miller, & S. M. Weiss (Eds.) *Behavioral health: A handbook on health enhancement and disease prevention.* (pp. 467–487). New York: Wiley.
Osborn, A. F. (1963). *Applied imagination.* New York: Scribner's.
Paffenberger, R. S., Hyde, R. T., Wing, A. L., & Steinmetz, E. H. (1984). A natural history of athleticism and cardiovascular health. *Journal of the American Medical Association, 252,* 491–495.
Peele, S. (1984). The cultural context of psychological approaches to alcoholism: Can we control the effects of alcohol? *American Psychologist, 39,* 1337–1351.
Pelletier, K. & Lutz, R. (1988). Healthy people, healthy business. *American Journal of Health Promotion, 2,* 5–12, 19.
Pennebaker, J. W. (1990). *Opening Up.* New York: William Morrow & Company.
Peterson, C., Seligman, M. P. E., & Vaillant, G. E. (1988). Pessimistic explanatory style is a risk factor for physical illness: A thirty-five-year longitudinal study. *Journal of Personality and Social Psychology, 55,* 23–27.
Premack, D. (1959). Toward empirical behavior laws: I. Positive reinforcement. *Psychological Review, 66,* 219–233.
President's Commission on Mental Health. (1978). *Report to the President.* Washington, DC: U.S. Government Printing Office.
Rama, Ballentine, R., & Ajaya. (1976). *Yoga and psychotherapy: The evolution of consciousness.* Glenview, IL: Himalayan Institute.
Rathus, S. A. (1973). A 30-item schedule for assessing assertive behavior. *Behavior Therapy, 4,* 398–406.
Robinson, D. (1979). *Talking out of alcoholism: The self-help process of Alcoholics Anonymous.* London: Croom, Helm.
Rosch, P. J. & Pelletier, K. R. (1987). Designing worksite stress management programs. In L. R. Murphy & T. F. Schoenborn (Eds.) *Stress management in work settings.* Washington, D. C. National Institute for Occupational Safety and Health. (pp. 69–91).
Rosen, G. M. (1982). Self-help approaches to self-management. In K. R. Blankstein & J. Polivy (Eds.), *Self-control and self-modification of emotional behavior* (pp. 183–199). New York: Plenum.
Roskies, E. (1983). Stress management: Averting the evil eye. *Contemporary Psychology, 28,* 542–544.
Russell, D., Cutrona, C. E., Rose, J., & Yurko, K. (1984). Social and emotional loneliness: An examination of Weiss's typology of loneliness. *Journal of personality and social psychology,* 46, 1313–1321.
Schachter, S. (1982). Recidivism and self-cure of smoking and obesity. *American Psychologist, 37,* 436–444.
Scheier, M. F. & Carver, C. S. (1987). Dispositional optimism and physical well-being: The influence of generalized outcome expectancies on health. *Journal of Personality, 55,* 169–210.
Schlegel, R. P., Wellwood, J. K., Copps, B. E., Gruchow, W. H., & Sharratt, M. T. (1980). The relationship between perceived challenge and daily symptom reporting in Type A vs. Type B postinfarct subjects. *Journal of Behavioral Medicine, 3,* 191–204.
Schneider, C. J. (1987). Cost effectiveness of biofeedback and behavioral medicine treatments: A review of the literature. *Biofeedback and Self-Regulation, 12,* 71–92.
Smith, J. C. (1991). *Stress Scripting: A guide to stress management.* New York: Praeger Publishers.
Smith, J. C. (1986). *Relaxation dynamics audiocassette series.* Champaign, IL: Research Press.
Smith, J. C. (1987). *Meditation: A sensible guide to a timeless discipline.* Champaign, IL: Research Press.
Smith, J. C. (1990). *Cognitive-behavioral relaxation training: A new system of strategies for treatment and assessment.* New York: Springer Publishing Company.
Smith, J. C. (1991a). *The Relaxation Wordlist.* Available from author. Chicago, IL
Smith, J. C. (1989). *Relaxation Dynamics: A cognitive-behavioral approach to relaxation.* Champaign, IL: Research Press.
Smith, J. C. (1992). *Spiritual living for a skeptical age: A psychological approach to meditative practice.* New York: Insight/Plenum.
Snyder, C. R., Harris, C., Anderson, J. R., Holleran, S. A., Irving, L. M., Sigmon, S. T., Yoshinobu, L., Gibb, J., Langelle, C., & Harnery, P. (1991). The will and the ways: Development and validation of an individual-differences measure of hope. *Journal of Personality and Social Psychology, 60,* 570–585.
Spache, G., & Berg, P. (1978). *The art of efficient reading* (3rd ed.). New York: Macmillan.
Spielberger, C. D., Gorsuch, R. C., & Lushene, R. E. (1970). *Manual for the State-Trait Anxiety Inventory.* Palo Alto: Consulting Psychologists.
Stachnik, T. J. & Stoffelmayr, B. E. (1983). Worksite smoking cessation programs: A potential for national impact. *American Journal of Public Health, 73,* 1395–1396.
Sternbach, R. A. (1987). *Mastering pain: A twelve-step program for coping with chronic pain.* New York: G. P. Putnam's Sons.
Stoyva, J. & Anderson, C. (1982). A coping-rest model of relaxation and stress management. In L. Goldberger & S. Breznitz (Eds.), *Handbook of stress: Theoretical and clinical aspects* (pp. 745–763). New York: Free Press.
Straw, M. K. (1983). Coping with obesity. In T. G. Burish & L. A. Bradley (Eds.)., *Coping with chronic disease: Research and applications* (pp. 219–258). New York: Academic Press.
Stunkard, A. J. (1975). From explanation to action in psychosomatic medicine: The case of obesity. *Psychosomatic Medicine, 37,* 195–236.
Stunkard, A. J. (1979). Behavioral medicine and beyond: The example of obesity. In O. F. Pomerleau and J. P. Brady (Eds.) *Behavioral medicine: Theory and practice.* Baltimore: Williams & Wilkins.
Taylor, S. E. (1989). *Positive illusions: Creative self-deception and the healthy mind.* New York: Basic Books.
Thoits, P. A. (1983). Dimensions of life events that influence psychological distress: An evaluation and synthesis of the literature. In Kaplan, H. B. (ed.) *Psychosocial stress: Trends in theory and research.* New York: Academic Press. pp. 33–103.
Thomas, E. I., & Robinson, H. A. (1982). *Improving reading in every class.* Boston: Allyn & Bacon.
Tomkins, S. (1966). Psychological model for smoking behavior. *American Journal of Public Health, 56* (12, Supplement), 17–20.
Tomkins, S. (1968). A modified model of smoking behavior. In E. F. Borgatta & R. R. Evans (Eds.). *Smoking, health and behavior.* Chicago, Aldine.
United States Public Health Service (1982). *The health consequences of smoking: Cancer. A report to the Surgeon General: 1982.* (Publication of Superintendent of Documents.) Washington, DC: U.S. Government Printing Office.
Walker, C. R. & Guest, R. H. (1952). *The man on the assembly line.* Cambridge, MA: Harvard University Press.
Warner, K. E. (1986). *Selling smoke: Cigarette advertising and public health.* Washington, DC: American Public Health Association.
Weissman, A. N. (1980). Assessing depressogenic attitudes: A validation study. Paper presented at the 51st Annual Meet-

ing of the Eastern Psychological Association, Hartford, CT.

Wilson, G. T. (1984). Weight control treatments. In J. D. Matarazzo, S. M. Weiss, J. A. Herd, N. E. Miller, & S. M. Weiss (Eds.) *Behavioral health: A handbook on health enhancement and disease prevention.* (pp. 657–670). New York: Wiley.

Wolpe, J. (1958). *Psychotherapy by reciprocal inhibition.* Stanford, CA: Stanford University Press.

Wright, R. A., Contrada, R. J., & Glass, D. C. (1985). Psychophysiologic correlates of Type A behavior. In Katkin, E. S. & Manuck, S. B. (eds.), *Advances in behavioral medicine.* Greenwich, Conn: JAI.

Zung, W. K. (1971). A rating instrument for anxiety disorders. *Psychosomatics, 12,* 371–379.

INDEX